Eating Disorders in Child and Adolescent Psychiatry

Editors

JAMES LOCK
JENNIFER DERENNE

CHILD AND ADOLESCENT PSYCHIATRIC CLINICS OF NORTH AMERICA

www.childpsych.theclinics.com

Consulting Editor
TODD E. PETERS

October 2019 • Volume 28 • Number 4

ELSEVIER

1600 John F. Kennedy Boulevard • Suite 1800 • Philadelphia, Pennsylvania, 19103-2899

http://www.theclinics.com

CHILD AND ADOLESCENT PSYCHIATRIC CLINICS OF NORTH AMERICA Volume 28, Number 4
October 2019 ISSN 1056–4993, ISBN-13: 978-0-323-67329-7

Editor: Lauren Boyle
Developmental Editor: Kristen Helm

Child and Adolescent Psychiatric Clinics of North America (ISSN 1056-4993) is published quarterly by Elsevier Inc., 360 Park Avenue South, New York, NY 10010-1710. Months of issue are January, April, July, and October. Business and Editorial Offices: 1600 John F. Kennedy Boulevard, Suite 1800, Philadelphia, PA 19103-2899. Periodicals postage paid at New York, NY and additional mailing offices. Subscription prices are $335.00 per year (US individuals), $627.00 per year (US institutions), $100.00 per year (US students), $388.00 per year (Canadian individuals), $762.00 per year (Canadian institutions), $200.00 per year (Canadian students), $446.00 per year (international individuals), $762.00 per year (international institutions), and $200.00 per year (international students). International air speed delivery is included in all *Clinics* subscription prices. All prices are subject to change without notice. **POSTMASTER:** Send address changes to *Child and Adolescent Psychiatric Clinics of North America*, Elsevier Health Sciences Division, Subscription Customer Service, 3251 Riverport Lane, Maryland Heights, MO 63043. **Customer Service: 1-800-654-2452 (U.S. and Canada); 314-447-8871 (outside U.S. and Canada). Fax: 314-447-8029. E-mail:** JournalsCustomer Service-usa@elsevier.com **(for print support)** or journalsonlinesupport-usa@elsevier.com **(for online support).**

Reprints. For copies of 100 or more of articles in this publication, please contact the Commercial Reprints Department, Elsevier Inc., 360 Park Avenue South, New York, New York 10010-1710 Tel.: 212-633-3874; Fax: 212-633-3820, E-mail: reprints@elsevier.com.

Child and Adolescent Psychiatric Clinics of North America is covered in *MEDLINE/PubMed (Index Medicus), ISI, SSCI, Research Alert, Social Search, Current Contents,* and *EMBASE/Excerpta Medica.*

Contributors

CONSULTING EDITOR

TODD E. PETERS, MD, FAPA
Medical Director, Child and Adolescent Services, Chief Medical Information Officer (CMIO), Sheppard Pratt Health System, Sheppard Pratt Physicians PA Clinical Operations Liaison, Baltimore, Maryland, USA

EDITORS

JAMES LOCK, MD, PhD
Professor of Psychiatry and Behavioral Sciences and Pediatrics, Division of Child and Adolescent Psychiatry, Associate Chair and Director, Eating Disorder Program, Stanford University School of Medicine, Stanford, California, USA

JENNIFER DERENNE, MD
Clinical Associate Professor of Psychiatry and Behavioral Sciences, Director of Inpatient Eating Disorders, Comprehensive Care Program, Division of Child and Adolescent Psychiatry, Stanford University School of Medicine, Psychiatry and Behavioral Sciences, Stanford, California, USA

AUTHORS

CARA BOHON, PhD
Assistant Professor, Department of Psychiatry and Behavioral Sciences, Stanford University School of Medicine, Stanford, California, USA

RACHEL BRYANT-WAUGH, BSc, MSc, DPhil
Honorary Senior Lecturer, Population, Policy and Practice Programme, UCL Great Ormond Street Institute of Child Health, London, United Kingdom

JENNIFER COUTURIER, MD, MSc
Associate Professor of Psychiatry, McMaster University, McMaster Children's Hospital, Hamilton, Ontario, Canada

KRISTEN M. CULBERT, PhD
Department of Psychology, University of Nevada, Las Vegas, Las Vegas, Nevada, USA

MARISA C. DeGUZMAN, BS, BA
Departments of Psychiatry and Neuroscience, University of Colorado Anschutz Medical Campus, School of Medicine, Children's Hospital Colorado, Aurora, Colorado, USA

JENNIFER DERENNE, MD
Clinical Associate Professor of Psychiatry and Behavioral Sciences, Director of Inpatient Eating Disorders, Comprehensive Care Program, Division of Child and Adolescent Psychiatry, Stanford University School of Medicine, Psychiatry and Behavioral Sciences, Stanford, California, USA

NATASHA FOWLER, MA
Department of Psychology, Michigan State University, East Lansing, Michigan, USA

GUIDO K.W. FRANK, MD
Professor in Psychiatry, University of California, San Diego, UCSD Eating Disorder Center, Rady Children's Hospital San Diego, San Diego, California, USA

SASHA GORRELL, PhD
Postdoctoral Clinical Psychology T32 Scholar, Department of Psychiatry, University of California, San Francisco, San Francisco, California, USA

LEANNA ISSERLIN, MD
Assistant Professor of Psychiatry, University of Ottawa, Children's Hospital of Eastern Ontario, Ottawa, Ontario, Canada

KELLY L. KLUMP, PhD
MSU Foundation Endowed Professor, Department of Psychology, Michigan State University, East Lansing, Michigan, USA

DANIEL LE GRANGE, PhD
Benioff UCSF Professor in Children's Health, Director, Department of Psychiatry, University of California, San Francisco, San Francisco, California, USA; Emeritus Professor of Psychiatry and Behavioral Neuroscience, The University of Chicago, Chicago, Illinois, USA

JAMES LOCK, MD, PhD
Professor of Psychiatry and Behavioral Sciences and Pediatrics, Division of Child and Adolescent Psychiatry, Associate Chair and Director, Eating Disorder Program, Stanford University School of Medicine, Stanford, California, USA

RUOFAN MA, BMath
Department of Psychology, Michigan State University, East Lansing, Michigan, USA

MEGAN E. MIKHAIL, BS
Department of Psychology, Michigan State University, East Lansing, Michigan, USA

STUART B. MURRAY, PhD
Department of Psychiatry, University of California, San Francisco, San Francisco, California, USA

MARK NORRIS, MD
Associate Professor of Pediatrics, University of Ottawa, Children's Hospital of Eastern Ontario, Ottawa, Ontario, Canada

REBECKA PEEBLES, MD
Director of Research and Quality Innovations, Eating Disorder Assessment and Treatment Program, The Children's Hospital of Philadelphia, Assistant Professor, Perelman School of Medicine, University of Pennsylvania, Roberts Center for Pediatric Research, Philadelphia, Pennsylvania, USA

SHIRI SADEH-SHARVIT, PhD
Baruch Ivcher School of Psychology, Interdisciplinary Center, Herzliya, Israel; Center for m²Health, Palo Alto University, Palo Alto, California, USA

MEGAN E. SHOTT, BS
University of California, San Diego, UCSD Eating Disorder Center, Rady Children's Hospital San Diego, San Diego, California, USA

ERIN HAYLEY SIEKE, MD, MS
Pediatric Resident Physician, The Children's Hospital of Philadelphia, Philadelphia, Pennsylvania, USA

WENDY SPETTIGUE, MD
Associate Professor of Psychiatry, University of Ottawa, Children's Hospital of Eastern Ontario, Ottawa, Ontario, Canada

Contents

> This article provides background information, descriptions, and evidential support for the more recent treatments for adolescents with anorexia nervosa, including family-based treatment, adolescent focused therapy, cognitive behavioral therapy, systemic family therapy, and psychopharmacologic treatments. At this time, family-based treatment has the best evidence of efficacy and cost-effectiveness. Future directions in treatment research for adolescent anorexia nervosa are discussed.

> There are few systematic studies of treatment of bulimia nervosa (BN) in adolescents. Although family-based treatment has demonstrated preliminary evidence to support involvement of caregivers in treatment, there is significant opportunity for improvement in mitigating binge-eating and purging symptoms among adolescents afflicted with BN. When caregivers are unable to participate in treatment, there is evidence that BN-specific cognitive behavioral therapy approaches are helpful for some adolescents. Further research is needed to determine for whom, and under what conditions certain types of family involvement might be most effective in adolescent treatment of BN.

> Binge eating disorder onset often occurs during adolescence, yet the diagnosis and treatment of the disorder in this age group has been inadequately studied. Criteria and challenges in making the diagnosis in children and adolescents are reviewed, as well as prevalence rates, current treatment options, and complications.

> Avoidant/restrictive food intake disorder (ARFID) is a relatively newly introduced diagnostic category within the feeding and eating disorders. This article summarizes current knowledge and clinical practice relating to ARFID in youth. It discusses epidemiology, diagnosis, clinical assessment, treatment interventions, prognosis, and outcome. Gaps in the existing research literature are highlighted, promising avenues of current research signposted, and potentially useful future directions proposed. The article is

relevant to clinicians wishing to ensure their practice is based on up-to-date information, as well as researchers interested in furthering knowledge relating to ARFID.

Eating disorders are common in children and adolescents, and may continue, resurface, or present anew in young people making the transition to adulthood. This may affect the young person's academic or occupational trajectory, and patients and parents/families need to recognize the supports that may be necessary to allow the emerging adult to be successful in navigating independent living, increased work or educational autonomy, and adult relationships. Colleges and universities are able to provide some support, but patients, families, and clinicians must be aware of limitations and must be thoughtful about options available to promote successful transition wherever possible.

Many eating disorder patients are successfully treated in outpatient settings. Family-based treatment allows youth to recover at home. Higher levels of care may be necessary for medical or psychiatric stabilization, or to provide added structure. Historically, hospital lengths of stay were long. Currently, insurance limitations encourage intermediate care levels to support patients not requiring inpatient treatment but not ready for outpatient care. Options include inpatient medical stabilization, locked units for individuals with suicidal ideation, and outpatient programs offering daily meal support and group therapy. Outpatient teams and families collaborate to determine the appropriate level of care.

Psychotropic medications are commonly used in the treatment of eating disorders in children and adolescents. This article reviews the evidence base on psychotropic medications, including all randomized trials, uncontrolled trials, and case reports for the treatment of anorexia nervosa, bulimia nervosa, other specified feeding and eating disorders, binge-eating disorder, and avoidant/restrictive food intake disorder. Despite advances in the number of medication-based studies completed in young patients with eating disorders over the last 2 decades, significantly more work needs to be done in terms of identifying what role, if any, psychotropic medications can have on treatment outcomes.

Eating disorders affect a significant number of individuals across the life span and are found among all demographic groups (including all genders, socioeconomic statuses, and ethnicities). They can cause malnutrition, which can have significant effects on every organ system in the body. Cardiovascular complications are particularly dangerous and cause eating disorders to have the highest mortality rate of all mental illnesses. This article outlines the medical assessment and treatment of malnutrition due to disordered eating.

Puberty is a critical risk period for eating disorders (EDs). ED incidence increases across the pubertal period and becomes female predominant, and genetic influences on disordered eating significantly increase. Surges of ovarian hormones, particularly estrogen, may drive this increasing genetic effect for EDs in pubertal girls and contribute to differential phenotypic presentations beyond puberty. In this article, we explain phenotypic associations between puberty and disordered eating and present evidence showing underlying genetic and hormonal influence. Potential benefits of communicating roles of genetic influence to people with or at risk for EDs are also discussed.

Eating disorders are severe psychiatric illnesses with a typical age of onset in adolescence. Brain research in youth and young adults may help us identify specific neurobiology that contributes to onset and maintenance of those disorders. This article provides a state-of-the-art review of our current understanding of the neurobiology of anorexia nervosa and bulimia nervosa. This includes brain structure and function studies to understand food restriction, binge-eating or purging behaviors, cognitive and emotional factors, as well as interoception. Binge-eating disorder and avoidant restrictive food intake disorder are also discussed, but the literature is still very small.

Eating disorders are serious psychiatric disorders, associated with significant psychiatric and medical consequences. Although traditionally considered a female disorder, more recent evidence has determined that EDs among males are not uncommon and are equally severe in symptom presentation. Among youth and adolescent males, certain factors increase the risk for ED, including muscularity-focused body image concerns and sexual orientation. Future study of these and other factors that may increase the risk for or maintain EDs among adolescent males is critical to improving screening, assessment, and precision treatment efforts.

Shiri Sadeh-Sharvit

For countless young people, technology plays an essential role in their lives. However, its many advantages have not yet been widely applied to the treatment of youth with eating disorders. This article looks at how smartphone applications, Web conferencing, and other developments could widen the range of care available in a field where suitable support can be hard to find. Various barriers to treatment exist, such as cost, access, and the stigma attached to eating disorders, but existing and new technologies could overcome those obstacles, if clinicians are willing and able to meet the requirements associated with digitally enhanced treatment.

CHILD AND ADOLESCENT PSYCHIATRIC CLINICS

ISSUE OF RELATED INTEREST

Psychiatric Clinics of North America
https://www.psych.theclinics.com/
Pediatric Clinics of North America
https://www.pediatric.theclinics.com/
Neurologic Clinics
https://www.neurologic.theclinics.com/

AACAP Members: Please go to www.jaacap.org for information on access to the Child and Adolescent Psychiatric Clinics. *Resident* Members of AACAP: Special access information is available at www.childpsych.theclinics.com.

THE CLINICS ARE AVAILABLE ONLINE!
Access your subscription at:
www.theclinics.com

CHILD AND ADOLESCENT PSYCHIATRIC CLINICS

FORTHCOMING ISSUES

January 2020
Psychosis in Children and Adolescents: A
Issue for Clinicians
Ellen M. House and John Tyson, Editors

April 2020
Autism Spectrum Disorder Across the
Lifespan: Part I
Thomas Flis, Scott R. Pekrul and Robert W.
Wisner-Carlson, Editors

July 2020
Autism Spectrum Disorder Across the
Lifespan: Part II
Thomas Flis, Scott R. Pekrul and Robert W.
Wisner-Carlson, Editors

RECENT ISSUES

July 2019
Depression in Special Populations
Warren Y.K. Ng and Karen Dineen
Wagner, Editors

April 2019
The Science of Well-Being: Integration into
Clinical Child Psychiatry
David Rettew, Matthew Biel, and Jeff
Bostic, Editors

January 2019
Reconsolidation in Child and Adolescent
Psychiatry
Jonathan Essery Becker, Christopher Todd
Maley, Elizabeth K.B. Shultz, and Todd E.
Peters, Editors

ISSUE OF RELATED INTEREST

Pediatric Clinics of North America
https://www.pediatric.theclinics.com
Pediatric Clinics of North America, Editor
https://www.pediatric.theclinics.com
Neurologic Clinics
https://www.neurologic.ps.theclinics.com

THE CLINICS ARE AVAILABLE ONLINE!

Access your subscription at:
www.theclinics.com

Preface

Treating Eating Disorders in Children and Adolescents: An Update

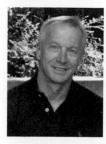 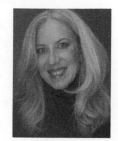

James Lock, MD, PhD   Jennifer Derenne, MD
Editors

It was a pleasure to edit this issue of *Child and Adolescent Psychiatric Clinics of North America* focused on eating disorders. Despite the fact that eating disorders retain the distinction of having the highest mortality of all mental illnesses, access to appropriate treatment remains problematic for many youth and their families. Outcomes data suggest that there is still much room for improvement, but ongoing research strives to better understand biological vulnerabilities to the illness, develop innovative treatments, and establish a strong evidence base to support those interventions.

Many child and adolescent psychiatrists feel underprepared to assess and make treatment recommendations for patients with eating disorders. All the same, with a relative dearth of subspecialty providers available, general child and adolescent psychiatrists are often asked to evaluate and treat these patients. They are also likely to encounter disordered eating in the context of their work with other patients; eating disorders are highly comorbid with mood, anxiety, obsessive compulsive disorders, substance use disorders, and personality disorders. Careful child and adolescent psychiatrists need to consider disordered eating when evaluating psychiatric symptoms that could be a manifestation of malnutrition.

For this reason, we decided to curate this issue of the *Child and Adolescent Psychiatric Clinics of North America* with an eye toward updating clinical recommendations for treating anorexia nervosa, bulimia nervosa, binge-eating disorder, and avoidant restrictive food intake disorder in children, adolescents, and transitional age youth. In addition to reviewing the evidence base for outpatient psychotherapeutic treatments, we include articles on higher levels of care, psychopharmacology in child and adolescent eating disorders, and a review of the medical complications of eating disorders as well as the assessment and treatment of malnutrition. We round out the

Child Adolesc Psychiatric Clin N Am 28 (2019) xiii–xiv
https://doi.org/10.1016/j.chc.2019.06.001
childpsych.theclinics.com
1056-4993/19/© 2019 Elsevier Inc. All rights reserved.

issue with articles on genetic contributions and the neurobiological basis for the development of eating disorders and conclude with a discussion of underrepresented populations (including male adolescents), and ways in which technology can be harnessed to aid in the successful treatment of eating disorders.

We are grateful to our contributing authors for sharing their research findings and clinical wisdom, and for the time and effort involved in this undertaking.

James Lock, MD, PhD
Psychiatry and Behavioral
Sciences and Pediatrics
Division of Child and
Adolescent Psychiatry
Eating Disorder Program
Stanford University School of Medicine
401 Quarry Road
MC 5719
Stanford, CA 94305, USA

Jennifer Derenne, MD
Psychiatry and Behavioral Sciences
Comprehensive Care Program
Division of Child and
Adolescent Psychiatry
Stanford University School of Medicine
401 Quarry Road
MC 5719
Stanford, CA 94305, USA

E-mail addresses:
jimlock@stanford.edu (J. Lock)
jderenne@stanford.edu (J. Derenne)

Updates on Treatments for Adolescent Anorexia Nervosa

James Lock, MD, PhD

KEYWORDS

- Anorexia nervosa • Adolescents • Treatments

KEY POINTS

- There have been significant advances in treatment of adolescents with anorexia nervosa (AN) over the past decade.
- Increasing evidence supports that family interventions, particularly those focused on parental behavioral management in the home environment (ie, family-based treatment [FBT]) are effective, efficient, and cost-effective. Other effective treatments include other forms of family therapy (eg, systemic family therapy) and a specific form of individual developmental and psychodynamic therapy (ie, adolescent-focused therapy).
- No new medication treatments have been identified that directly treat AN.
- A range of adaptations to FBT may improve recovery rates that currently hover between 40% and 50%.
- Further research to identify new treatments for AN is needed.

INTRODUCTION

Anorexia nervosa (AN) is serious eating disorder, typically with onset in early adolescence. It is characterized by dramatic weight loss, usually resulting from a combination of severe food restriction and overexercise. These behaviors

---

Disclosure: The author receives royalties for manuals describing family-based treatment from Guilford Press and Routledge. The author receives consultation and training compensation from the Training Institute of Child and Adolescent Eating Disorders.
Department of Psychiatry and Behavioral Sciences, Stanford University, 401 Quarry Road, Stanford, CA 94305, USA
E-mail address: jimlock@stanford.edu

Child Adolesc Psychiatric Clin N Am 28 (2019) 523–535
https://doi.org/10.1016/j.chc.2019.05.001
1056-4993/19/© 2019 Elsevier Inc. All rights reserved.

childpsych.theclinics.com

are accompanied by obsessive preoccupations and fears about weight gain, appearance, and food. This combination of behavioral and psychological characteristics leads to a full range of emotional, behavioral, social, and familial impairments. AN is associated with one of the highest mortality rates of all psychiatric illnesses.[1] Death results from the physiologic impact of malnutrition, particularly related to cardiovascular dysrhythmia.[2] Nonetheless, the psychological toll is also substantial and leads to a significant proportion of patients dying by suicide.[3] Contrary to stereotypes of AN occurring only in rich white females, AN occurs in persons across the gender spectrum, and in all racial, ethnic, and socioeconomic groups. AN has a prevalence of 0.5% to 1.5% in young women.[4] Current estimates suggest that the ratio of females to males is 10:1.[5,6]

AN is a very old psychiatric disorder with medical descriptions going back to Richard Morton[7] in 1689 in a case series of what he called nervous consumption. In 1874, William Gull[8] was the first to describe the clinical syndrome comprehensively and the first to call it AN. He identified the principle diagnostic features of self-starvation and weight preoccupation, which characterize all diagnostic formulations of AN to this day. Although some of the details have changed, the conception and fundamental characteristics of AN have not changed much over time. In this sense, it is among most enduring psychiatric formulations. Furthermore, data suggest that the disorder occurs cross-culturally,[9] with few differences in clinical presentation, though weight phobia may be less pronounced in some Asian populations.[10]

The causes of AN are unknown. There is clearly a heritable component to the disorder. Family aggregation studies find AN is 5 times more common in families with another first-degree relative with an eating disorder than those without. Heritability estimates based on twin studies range from 30% to 75% in AN.[11] Furthermore, 1 study found that for prepubertal twins genetic influences were not significant.[12] However, for older twins, heritability was high.[13] One proposed mechanism to explain this gene and development interaction is that hormonal changes occurring during puberty mediate gene expression.[14,15] Temperamental variables have also been implicated in the cause of AN, particularly perfectionistic, obsessive, and avoidant features, which are also likely heritable.[11,16–18] Recent studies also suggest that heritable cognitive styles related to detail processing and flexible thinking could be a cause of AN.[19–23]

In addition to biologically based theories, others have proposed that AN is the result of fear or avoidance of adolescent development, including physical, psychosexual, and family factors. Arthur Crisp[24,25] is perhaps the leading proponent of this theory; however, it shares theoretic underpinnings with the theories of inadequate self-esteem, confidence, and assertiveness found in the work of Hilde Bruch.[26,27] Others have suggested that family dysfunction or pathologic conditions underlie the disorder,[28] but there is no substantive evidence to support these claims. At the same time, others have suggested that social and cultural factors related to the promotion of the thin ideal in the media are possible causative factors.[29–31] In addition, trauma (physical and sexual) are proposed causes. Participation in activities such as modeling, gymnastics, ballet, and wrestling seem to increase the risk for developing AN, presumably because appearance and/or weight directly affect performance or assessment of performance.[30,32] Over all, little data currently support the specificity of any of the putative causes AN; therefore, explaining the cause of AN remains impossible.

CLINICAL PRESENTATION

> *Maggie is a 14-year-old female who began dieting about 6 months ago. She has increasing narrowed both the amount and types of food she will eat. She began by eliminating desserts, then breads, but has now become a vegetarian. She drinks only water and claims foods that contain sugar, fat, or gluten make her nauseous. However, she spends many hours in the kitchen and bakes cookies and cakes for her family even though she refuses to eat them. Maggie also has greatly increased her exercise. She runs at least 5 miles every day but usually more. In addition, she does several hundred stomach crunches every day. If she is unable to complete her workout, she is distraught. These activities and preoccupations have led to her spending less and less time with her peers. Though her academic work remains stellar, she now insists on standing while she does her homework. Maggie has lost more than 20 pounds in the last 3 months but feels she is still fat. Her pediatrician has noted that her heart rate and blood pressure are dropping. She checks her appearance in mirrors and store windows, often pulling up her shirt to pinch the fat on her abdomen. She is no longer menstruating. Maggie wears baggy clothes and reports feeling cold even when the rest of the family is comfortable. Maggie has become hard to live with. In the past, she was a compliant child, but now she is easily annoyed and becomes irritated and agitated, especially at mealtimes.*

As this case illustrates, the cardinal features of AN are fear of weight gain; obsessive preoccupation with food, weight, and exercise; and distorted body image; that is, feeling fat even though clearly emaciated (**Box 1**). However, in addition to these characteristics, a key element to the presentation of AN is that the symptoms are experienced as egosyntonic; that is, the person with AN wants to continue in her or his concerning behaviors despite the medical, psychiatric, and social consequences. This means that there is little or no motivation for treatment. As a result, engaging and retaining a patient with AN in treatment is a central problem.

TREATMENT APPROACHES FOR ANOREXIA NERVOSA IN YOUTH
Hospitalization

From the earliest medical descriptions from Gull,[8] Lasegue, and Charcot, hospitalization had been a recommended treatment of AN. The rationale that these early clinicians made for this was based on the belief that the parents of those afflicted with AN had pathologic tendencies. Charcot was unapologetic for his recommendation

---

Box 1
Clinical features of anorexia nervosa

- Severe dieting and/or excessive exercise, leading to inadequate nutrition to meet energy needs
- Clinically significant weight loss or not achieving expected growth
- Expressed fear or persistent behaviors (eg, severe dieting or excessive exercise) that prevent weight gain or expected growth
- Lack of concern or denial about malnutrition or body image distortion (believing one is fat when one is emaciated)
- AN can result from restriction and overexercise alone, or include episodes of binge eating and/or purging (ie, binge eating or purging subtype).

for hospitalization and believed that it was necessary to avert what he called the pernicious influence of parents.[33] However, the success of hospital treatment has not lived up to the theory. The 2 major studies that examined the use of specialized hospitalization programs for AN compared with outpatient treatments failed to find differential benefit of the approach despite the intensity and costs of such programs.[34,35] These studies do not suggest there is no role for hospitalization for AN but that, overall, hospitalization conveyed no systematic benefit compared with outpatient treatment. Thus, who will benefit from specialized hospitalization programs remains a vexing unanswered question.

Current hospitalization for AN is of 2 types:

1. Hospitalization to stabilize the acute medical problems associated with malnutrition that results from weight loss in AN.
2. Psychiatric hospitalization for continued weight gain beyond that necessary for acute medical problems and for changing the maintaining behaviors and cognitions of AN.

Weight loss and malnutrition in AN are associated with many medical problems, including but not limited to: bradycardia, prolonged QT_c, dysthymia, amenorrhea, electrolyte abnormalities, hypothermia, refeeding syndrome (rare but potentially life-threatening phosphate and magnesium decreases), osteopenia, and osteoporosis. The use of acute medical hospitalization for cardiac abnormalities, orthostasis, hypothermia, electrolyte abnormalities, and the prevention of refeeding syndrome is a medical necessity. Current indications for acute hospital treatment of these medical problems are available and summarized in **Table 1**.[36] These criteria are based on consensus guidelines rather than on a strong evidence base, but they represent the current best practice. Hospital programs using these criteria typically have a behaviorally oriented milieu that supports safe nutritional intake, rest, and psychoeducation of the patient and the family. Some programs use overnight tube feeding with the goal of decreasing length of stay, but little evidence supports substantive benefits of this approach. Clear guidelines for the most effective approach are lacking, but recent studies suggest that more rapid refeeding protocols are likely safe and would decrease medical stays.[37] Behavioral protocols vary widely. Some encourage patient management of intake (using menus from which the patients choose their meals) and others are prescriptive. With the advent of increasing parental involvement in the care of adolescents with AN (see later discussion of family-based treatment [FBT]), many programs are focusing on parental education about diet and nutrition and encouraging learning from nursing staff about successful

Table 1	
Main criteria for medical hospitalization for adolescents with anorexia nervosa	
Cardiac	Pulse <50 beats/min at daytime, <45 beats/min at night Prolonged QT_c >460 ms
Blood Pressure (BP)	Hypotension: BP <90/45 mm Hg Orthostasis: pulse increase >20 beats/min; systolic BP decrease >20 mm Hg; diastolic BP decrease >10 mm Hg
Body Temperature	T <35.6°C/96°F
Body Mass Index	<75% median body mass index for age and sex

Modified from Golden NH, Katzman DK, Sawyer SM, et al. Update on the medical management of eating disorders in adolescents. J Adolesc Health 2015;56(4):372; with permission.

approaches to helping their children at home when they are discharged. Most programs that treat adolescents with AN for acute medical problems expect a length of stay between 1 to 4 weeks, depending on the degree and rate of weight loss before being admitted.

Regarding psychiatric inpatient treatment of adolescent AN, there is less clarity about the best practices for such programs. The clinical goals and programmatic elements vary widely from specialty center to center. Some use behavioral and cognitive approaches, others emphasize individuation and adolescent development, and still others use elements of dialectic behavioral therapy. Almost all programs aim to foster weight restoration through regularizing intake and diet management, usually through professional dieticians. As mentioned previously, the data supporting the systematic efficacy of these specialized programs are quite limited, but what data are available do not suggest it is necessary or differentially beneficial for most adolescent patients.[38,39] Although there is little doubt that some patients need and benefit from such programs, the lack of a clear consensus on who will benefit and what type of inpatient psychiatric treatment is most effective remains a major problem for clinicians who treat adolescents with AN. However, it should be acknowledged that, even if who would respond and what kinds of inpatient treatment would be best were identified, there should be no expectation that inpatient psychiatric treatment will be sufficient or even adequate for treatment of adolescent AN. Basic learning principles related to generalization of learning contend that, for learning to be generalized, it must be practiced in the environment in which the skills and behaviors will be used. Hospitals, no matter how sensitively designed, are not generalizable environments. Thus, the expectation that what patients learn and can manage behaviorally in that setting will be transferred to their home environment is unrealistic. This explains why, after such hospitalization, most of the weight gain and behavioral changes accomplished rapidly decrease in the first few weeks after discharge, resulting in high rates of rehospitalization. It is clear that even when there is an effective program to help with weight restoration and related behaviors and cognitions, it is necessary for an effective outpatient approach if adolescents with AN who are hospitalized are to continue to improve.

Other Intensive Treatment Programs for Adolescent Anorexia Nervosa

There are myriad other intensive program that are designed to treat adolescents with AN, including partial hospitalization programs, afterschool programs, and residential programs. Sometimes, these programs are conceived of as either a kind of step-down from an inpatient psychiatric or medical program to assist with the transition to home or as a strategy to intervene early to prevent the necessity of admission to an inpatient program. Other times, they are conceived of as an alternative to outpatient or inpatient treatment; this is particularly the case for residential programs. Unfortunately, there is little systematic evidence that these programs are effective in achieving any of these goals. In many places, such programs have replaced inpatient psychiatric programs as an insurance-supported alternative to higher cost hospitalization. Most of these programs are proprietary and for-profit.[40] Studies about the effectiveness of these programs are likely biased in terms of population studies (insured and accepted to the program), nonsystematic follow-up data (many potential and former patients do not provide data), no randomization to comparison treatments, and potential publication bias due to a possible impact on program financial sustainability.[41,42] These comments do not mean that all such program are not helpful or that no one should or could benefit from them, but the evidence base supporting them as an effective and/or cost-effective treatment is absent.

Outpatient Psychosocial Treatments for Adolescent Anorexia Nervosa

In many ways, it is remarkable that there are such profoundly limited data related to treatment efficacy in AN.[43] As noted, this disorder has been identified for well over a hundred years. There are many possible reasons for this, including a long period when little systematic research on treatments for psychiatric disorders was conducted. When research began, many studies were pharmacologic (see later discussion), but these were not promising and this may have contributed to a general lack of enthusiasm among researchers to examine treatments for AN. The advent of psychosocial research based on cognitive behavioral therapy (CBT) for depression and anxiety ushered in the possibility that a modified version of this form of psychotherapy might useful for AN. Studies initially focused on bulimia nervosa and demonstrated efficacy of other approaches (eg, medications) for this disorder.[44] For AN, though, CBT seemed to be less effective in early trials.[45,46] One reason for the lack of response to CBT and other psychosocial treatments may have been that these early studies focused on the most difficult patients with AN: adults with an enduring and persistent AN.[47] In retrospect, this seems peculiar in many ways, including that most of these patients began their illnesses as adolescents. However, they were often a convenient sample, living for long periods of time in hospitals. None of the early studies recruited or studied adolescents with systematic treatments.

Over the past several decades, however, there has been an increase in the quantity and quality of studies for adolescents with AN, which has allowed the development of a fledgling database to inform clinical practice.[48] There are now 11 randomized clinical trials (RCTs) encompassing more than a 1000 participants published since 1987.[49] These are still small numbers in the big picture, to be sure, but they have nonetheless yielded important evidence that is useful for current clinical practice.[3] Most of these studies examined family therapy as 1 arm of the study, so the most extensive evidence is for a specific form of family therapy, FBT, which was manualized first in 2001, allowing subsequent use in studies and dissemination and implementation.[50] Other approaches, such as a specific form of individual therapy called adolescent-focused therapy (AFT),[51] CBT,[38] and systemic family therapy,[52] also have evidential support, though less so than FBT.

Currently, FBT is the treatment that has the largest evidence base for the treatment of adolescent AN and is recognized as the first-line approach by many national and international guidelines (https://www.nice.org.uk/guidance/ng69).[53] The approach helps parents and families disrupt the behaviors (ie, self-starvation, overexercise, persistent weight checks, body checking) that maintain AN in their homes. Thus, therapists help parents learn to do at home (a generalizable learning environment unlike hospitals or day or residential programs) what nurses and other professional staff do in intensive settings. The therapy aims to educate, empower, and support parents in specific techniques to address the need for parents working together, setting specific goals for behavior change, using consistent and persistent management strategies, curtailing negotiating behaviors, and minimizing emotional responses to demands and protesting verbal and physical behaviors. Therapists help parents to use their own skills and parenting strategies that have been stymied by AN and to adopt new ones, as needed, to address AN. The treatment has 3 phases. The first phase is focused on helping parent learn how to take charge and change the maintaining behaviors of AN, such that their child begins to gain weight under their supervision. This phase usually lasts about 3 months. Phase 2 begins when weight is mostly restored and allows for a gradual age-appropriate transition of control of eating and exercise back to their child. This phase allows the child to demonstrate sufficient mastery of these behaviors to allow them to eat with progressive independence. This phase usually lasts about 2 to 3 months. Phase 3 begins when the child is eating is sufficient for health and growth without the parents having to intervene. The aim of this brief phase is to transition the child and family back to normal adolescent developmental process. The focus is no longer on AN but on the impact of AN on adolescent development and ways to reenter this normal developmental process. This phase usually lasts 1 to 2 months. Thus FBT usually lasts between 10 to 20 sessions over 6 to 12 months.

An alternative family treatment to FBT is manualized systemic family therapy (SyFT).[52] This approach has been studied in only 1 outpatient clinical trial to date, but it was as effective as FBT, though slower to achieve treatment effects and significantly more costly because more patients needed inpatient treatment.[54] This approach is distinguished from FBT because it focuses on the general family process and changing unhelpful interactions and communication patterns in the family rather than on changing eating-related specific behaviors in the child. SyFT also has 3 phases. The first phase is devoted to building the therapeutic trust and relationship with the therapist and collecting information about current interaction and communication styles with an eye to both strengths and problems. Once these are identified, phase 2 can begin, in which the focus is on asking the family to evaluate and challenge the interactions they find unhelpful and wish to change. The third phase is aimed at helping the family experiment with trying new interactions and communication strategies. SyFT typically consists of between 10 to 20 sessions over 6 to 12 months.

Individual therapeutic approaches have been a mainstay of AN treatment. These are often rooted in either CBT approaches or developmental and psychodynamic theories. As noted previously, there are little data available on CBT for adolescents with AN. A small study in a residential treatment program in Italy reports preliminary data that suggest it may be feasible,[55] whereas a large RCT in the United Kingdom found CBT to be as effective as other treatments offered (inpatient and general outpatient care).[38] However, at this point, CBT for adolescent AN remains largely untested.

Two studies have examined the use of a developmentally informed individual psychodynamic treatment of adolescent AN.[56,57] The first study was relatively small and compared this form of individualized treatment to a form of FBT. Patients did well in both groups but, overall, did better in FBT. In a larger study of individualized AFT, it did about as well as FBT at the end of treatment, albeit more slowly and at a higher cost owing to more hospitalization. Over time, however, adolescents who received FBT had higher recovery rates. Nonetheless, AFT is likely best considered the second-best evidence-based approach for adolescent AN.

Similar to FBT and SyFT, AFT has 3 phases. There is a published description of the approach, but no detailed manual is yet available.[51] Treatment usually includes between 15 to 20 individual session with the adolescent, plus 5 to 8 sessions with parents over a 9 to 12 month period. The first phase is focused on building a therapeutic alliance, which is essential in this form of therapy.[58] It is also an opportunity for the therapist to gather the clinical information necessary to identify the central developmental, relational, or emotional challenge the adolescent is using AN to manage. At the heart of AFT is the idea that the undereating, overcontrol of eating, overexercise, and excessive focus on weight and shape are strategies that help the adolescent manage emotions and avoid challenging developmental challenges. At the end of phase 1, the therapist has identified the core problems. In phase 2, the therapist begins to help the adolescent learn how to manage these problems without resorting to the behaviors and preoccupations of AN. During this phase, the adolescent is required to eat enough to maintain and gain weight through direct counseling on the need for this by the therapist or, in some instances, through counseling by other professionals (eg, pediatricians, registered dieticians, nurses). The third phase is focused on consolidation and practice of strategies to cope with emotions and relationships, and on termination with the therapist. Collateral sessions with the parents are designed for the therapist to help the parents support their child's development and support exploration and experimentation related to adolescence.

Psychopharmacology of Adolescent Anorexia Nervosa

There are no medications approved by the US Food and Drug Administration for the treatment of AN. Furthermore, there is no systematic support for any pharmacologic agent efficacy for adolescents with AN. Several small to medium-sized RCTs have been conducted exploring both antidepressants[59] and atypical antipsychotics,[60] but the results of these studies have not provided clear support for efficacy.[61,62] Thus, the use of medications for adolescent AN is experimental and should typically be considered for the acute management of behavioral or emotional agitation that cannot be contained through behavioral management techniques or for comorbid psychiatric conditions. However, there are challenges with the use of medication in both these situations. Use of atypical antipsychotics for acute agitation requires care and usually very low doses in these usually medically fragile patients. Furthermore, this use should be discontinued after the agitation is sufficiently under control to reduce the chances of unwanted side effects and to clarify to the treatment team and parents that the medication is being used specifically in this temporizing manner and is not meant to be seen as effective for the symptoms of AN.

In the case of using medication for comorbid conditions, other problems can arise. When adolescents present with AN, they are often severely underweight, unhappy, irritable, obsessive, and anxious. Many would, therefore, qualify at the time of presentation for a range comorbid conditions, including anxiety disorders, depression, and obsessive-compulsive disorder. However, in many cases, these symptoms are expressions of AN rather than separate disorders. The exception to this is when there is a clear history of these diagnoses before the onset of AN. In those instances, prescribing or continuing to prescribe medications for the comorbid condition may be indicated, even during the acute early treatment period. However, in most presentations, there is no documented history of comorbid disorders. In those cases, it is best to treat AN first and only after there is a reasonable response to treatment (ie, weight gain to near normal weight range and decreased eating-related obsessional thoughts and behaviors) and the continued presence of symptoms consistent with a true comorbid diagnosis, would prescribing medication for this second disorder be indicated. Prescribing medications too early may render them less effective (serotonin supplies and reserves may be low) and may also risk focusing treatment on these possible other disorders rather than on AN.

New Possibilities in Treating Adolescents with Anorexia Nervosa

As noted at the outset, there is a long way to go in finding effective treatments for adolescents with AN. Several strategies may help us improve the outcomes of these patients. For example, existing effective treatments could be augmented or improved. In the case of FBT, data suggest that a clear marker of early response is a strong predictor of long-term recovery.[63] Specifically, by about 4 weeks of treatment, weight gain of about 5 pounds predicts recovery in about 80% of cases, whereas failure to achieve this milestone means recovery rates drop by 30%. So, developing and targeting a treatment that will enhance response rates in those who do not respond early is a possible way forward. A treatment to do just that has been developed and piloted that has demonstrated feasibility and preliminary data supporting likely efficacy. This approach, called intensive parental coaching (IPC),[64] is now being tested in a large multisite trial. An important finding related to improving early response is the identification of a possible mechanism of the approach. It seems that, in those for whom FBT is most effective, there is a robust change in this parental self-efficacy early in treatment (before weight gain).[65,66] Thus, one of the goals of IPC is to invigorate parental self-efficacy.

Another strategy is to identify those at risk of not responding to FBT at baseline. One of the consistent findings in the FBT literature is that obsessive-compulsive thinking is a predictor or moderator of poorer response.[54] The presence of a high degree of this type of thinking may make it more difficult for parents to be successful at challenging the maintaining behaviors of AN during FBT. Also, as previously noted, perseverative, rigid, and overly detailed thinking styles (neglecting the big picture) are common in patients with AN.[20,67] Adding a treatment to address these thinking styles might be a way to enhance response. Preliminary data suggest that cognitive remediation therapy, which is designed to do this, is acceptable and feasible to adolescents with AN, and can be added to FBT.[68] Further study is required to determine whether adding this approach to standard FBT will improve response rates.

FBT has mostly been studied in whole family formats; that is, the entire family meets with the therapist in sessions. However, 2 pilot studies and 1 reasonably scaled RCT suggest that seeing the parents alone may be as or even more effective than seeing the entire family.[69,70] Because family emotional climate (expressed emotion or family criticism) is a possible predictor or poor treatment response in FBT,[69] this change in format may be particularly helpful for families in which there are high levels of family criticism. Another change in format for FBT moves in the opposite direction: seeing groups of families together.[71,72] Studies suggest that some families find this approach supportive and combats the isolation associated with AN treatment. Data on the effectiveness of the approach remain limited.[71]

Other than trying to improve FBT through the strategies previously described, new approaches are needed for those who do not or cannot use FBT. As noted, AFT may be a reasonable second-line option. It the treatment study comparing AFT to FBT, those with less psychopathology, defined by lower Eating Disorder Examination scores, lower obsessions and compulsions related to eating, and without binge eating or purging, did just as well in AFT as FBT.[73] It would be useful to examine and confirm this finding to help match patients to this treatment when desired. Furthermore, refinement of AFT to identify ways to increase the efficiency of the approach (ie, lowering the dose) while also decreasing hospitalization would be important next steps. Similarly, exploring for whom CBT might be useful among adolescents with AN through further study of this approach in this younger age group is needed. For SyFT, additional studies are needed to confirm the finding that this approach is effective. Like AFT, however, the treatment needs refinement to improve efficiencies and cost-effectiveness.

SUMMARY

There have been significant advances in treatment of adolescents with AN over the past decade. Increasing evidence supports that family interventions, particularly those focused on parental behavioral management in the home environment (ie, FBT), are effective, efficient, and cost-effective. Other effective treatments include other forms of family therapy (ie, SyFT) and a specific form of individual developmental and psychodynamic therapy (ie, AFT). No new medication treatments have been identified that directly treat AN. A range of adaptations to FBT may improve recovery rates that currently hover between 40% and 50%. Further research to identify new treatments for AN is needed.

REFERENCES

1. Crow S, Peterson C, Swanson S, et al. Increased mortality in bulimia nervosa and other eating disorders. Am J Psychiatry 2009;166:1342–6.
2. Jauregui-Garrido B, Jauregui-Lobera I. Sudden death in eating disorders. Vasc Health Risk Management 2012;8:91–8.
3. Lock JL, LaVia M. Practice parameter for the assessment and treatment of children and adolescents with eating disorders. J Am Acad Child Adolesc Psychiatry 2015;54(5):412–25.
4. Smink FR, van Hoeken D, Oldehinkel AJ, et al. Prevalence and severity of DSM-5 eating disorders in a community cohort of adolescents. Int J Eat Disord 2014; 47(6):610–9.
5. Lock J. Fitting square pegs in round holes: males with eating disorders. J Adolesc Health 2008;2:99–100.
6. Hatchman G. Boys with eating disorders. J Sch Nurs 2005;6:329–32.
7. Morton R. Phthisiologia: or, a treatise of consumptions. London: Smith & Walford; 1694.
8. Gull W. Anorexia nervosa (apepsia hysterica, anorexia hysterica). Trans Clin Soc Lond 1874;7:222–8.
9. Smink F, van hoeken D, Hoek H. The epidemiology of eating disorders: incidence, prevalence, and mortality rates. Curr Psychiatry Rep 2012;14:406–14.
10. Lee H, Lock J. Anorexia nervosa in Asian-Americans: do they differ from their non-Asian peers. Int J Eat Disord 2007;40:227–31.
11. Bulik C, Sullivan P, Tozzi F, et al. Prevalence, heritability and prospective risk factors for anorexia nervosa. Arch Gen Psychiatry 2006;63:305–12.
12. Klump KL, McGue M, Iacona W. Age differences in genetic and environmental influences on eating attitudes and behaviors in preadolescent female twins. J Abnorm Psychol 2000;109:239–51.
13. Klump KL, Burt SA, McGue M, et al. Changes in genetic and environmental influences on disordered eating across adolescence: a longitudinal twin study. Arch Gen Psychiatry 2007;64:1409–15.
14. Klump KL, McGue M, Iacona W. Differential heritability of eating attitudes and behaviors in prepubertal versus pubertal twins. Int J Eat Disord 2003;33:287–92.
15. Klump KL, Perkins P, Burt SA, et al. Puberty moderates genetic influences on disordered eating. Psychol Med 2007;37:627–34.
16. Klump K, Bulik CM, Pollice C, et al. Temperament and character in women with anorexia nervosa. J Nerv Ment Dis 2000;188:559–67.
17. Cassin S, von Ramson L. Personality and eating disorders: a decade in review. Clin Psychol Rev 2005;25:895–916.
18. Wade T, Tiggemann M, Bulik CM, et al. Shared temperament risk factors for anorexia nervosa: a twin study. Psychosom Med 2008;70:239–44.
19. Tchanturia K, Davies H, Harrison A, et al. Poor cognitive flexibility in eating disorders: examining the evidence. PLoS One 2012;7:e28331.

20. Lopez C, Tchanturia K, Stahl D, et al. Central coherence in eating disorders: a systematic review. Psychol Med 2008;38:1075–84.
21. Holliday J, Tchanturia K, Landau S, et al. Is impaired set-shifting an endophenotype of anorexia nervosa? Am J Psychiatry 2005;162:2269–75.
22. Treasure J. Getting beneath the phenotype of anorexia nervosa: the search for viable endophenotypes and genotypes. Can J Psychiatry 2007;52:212–9.
23. Fitzpatrick K, Lock J, Darcy A, et al. Neurocognitive processes in adolescent anorexia nervosa. 2012:12. doi:2010.1002/eat.22027.
24. Crisp AH. Anorexia nervosa: let me be. London: Academic Press; 1980.
25. Crisp AH. Anorexia nervosa as flight from growth: assessment and treatment based on the model. In: Garner DM, Garfinkel P, editors. Handbook of treatment for eating disorders. New York: Guilford; 1997. p. 248–77.
26. Bruch H. Eating disorders: obesity, anorexia nervosa, and the person within. New York: Basic Books; 1973.
27. Bruch H. The golden cage: the enigma of anorexia nervosa. Cambridge (MA): Harvard University Press; 1978.
28. Minuchin S, Rosman B, Baker I. Psychosomatic families: anorexia nervosa in context. Cambridge (MA): Harvard University Press; 1978.
29. Field A. Risk factors for eating disorders: an evaluation of the evidence. In: Thompson JK, editor. Handbook of eating disorders and obesity. Hoboken (NJ): John Wiley & Sons; 2004. p. 17–32.
30. Anderson-Fye, Becker AE. Sociocultural aspects of eating disorders. In: Thompson J, editor. Handbook of eating disorders and obesity. Hoboken (NJ): John Wiley & Sons; 2004. p. 565–89.
31. Levine M, Harrison K. Media's role in the perpetuation and prevention of negative body image and disordered eating. In: Thompson J, editor. Handbook of eating disorders and obesity. Hoboken (NJ): John Wiley & Sons; 2004. p. 695–717.
32. Stice E. Sociocultural influences on body image and eating disturbance. In: Fairburn CG, Brownell K, editors. Eating and weight disorders and obesity: a comprehensive handbook. 2nd edition. New York: Guilford Press; 2002. p. 103–7.
33. Silverman J. Charcot's comments on the therapeutic role of isolation in the treatment of anorexia nervosa. Int J Eat Disord 1997;21:295–8.
34. McKenzie JM. Hospitalization for anorexia nervosa. Int J Eat Disord 1992;11:235–41.
35. Zhao Y, Encinosa W. Hospitalizations for Eating Disorders from 1999 to 2006. HCUP Statistical Brief #70. Rockville, MD: Agency for Healthcare Research and Quality; 2009. http://www.hcup-us.ahrq.gov/reports/statbriefs/sb70.pdf.
36. Golden NH, Katzman DK, Sawyer SM, et al. Update on the medical management of eating disorders in adolescents. J Adolesc Health 2015;56(4):370–5.
37. Garber A, Sawyer S, Golden N, et al. A systematic review of approaches to refeeding inpatients with anorexia nervosa. Int J Eat Disord 2016;49(3):293–310.
38. Gowers S, Clark A, Roberts C, et al. Clinical effectiveness of treatments for anorexia nervosa in adolescents. Br J Psychiatry 2007;191(5):427–35.
39. Crisp AH, Norton K, Gowers S, et al. A controlled study of the effect of therapies aimed at adolescent and family psychopathology in anorexia nervosa. Br J Psychiatry 1991;159:325–33.
40. Frisch J, Franko D, Herzog DB. Residential treatment for eating disorders. Int J Eat Disord 2006;39:434–9.
41. Brewerton T, Costin C. Treatment results of anorexia nervosa and bulimia nervosa in a residential treatment program. Eat Disord 2011;19:117–31.

42. Brewerton T, Costin C. Long-term outcome of residential treatment for anorexia nervosa and bulimia nervosa. Eat Disord 2011;19:132–44.
43. Bulik CM, Berkman N, Kimberly A, et al. Anorexia nervosa: a systematic review of randomized clinical trials. Int J Eat Disord 2007;40:310–20.
44. Fairburn C. A cognitive behavioural approach to the treatment of bulimia. Psychol Med 1981;11(4):707–11.
45. Pike K, Walsh BT, Vitousek K, et al. Cognitive-behavioral therapy in the posthospitalization treatment of anorexia nervosa. Am J Psychiatry 2004;160:2046–9.
46. McIntosh VW, Jordan J, Carter FA, et al. Three psychotherapies for anorexia nervosa: a randomized, controlled trial. Am J Psychiatry 2005;162:741–7.
47. Hay PJ, Touyz S, Sud R. Treatment for severe and enduring anorexia nervosa: a review. Aust N Z J Psychiatry 2012. https://doi.org/10.1177/0004867412450469 2012.
48. Lock J. An update on evidence based psychosocial interventions for children and adolescents with eating disorders. J Clin Child Adolesc Psychol 2015;44:707–21.
49. Lock J. Family therapy for eating disorders in youth: current confusions, advances, and new directions. Curr Opin Psychiatry 2018;31(6):431–5.
50. Lock J, Le Grange D. Treatment manual for anorexia nervosa: a family-based approach. 2nd edition. New York: Guilford Press; 2013.
51. Fitzpatrick K, Moye A, Hostee R, et al. Adolescent focused therapy for adolescent anorexia nervosa. J Contemp Psychother 2010;40:31–9.
52. Pote H, Stratton P, Cottrell D, et al. Systemic family therapy manual. 2001. Available at: http://www.psyc.leeds.ac.uk/research/lftrc/intro_mtap.htm. Accessed August 1, 2001.
53. Hilbert A, Hoek H, Schmidt R. Evidence-based clinical guidelines for eating disorders: international comparison. Curr Opin Psychiatry 2017;30:423–37.
54. Agras W, Lock J, Brandt H, et al. Comparison of 2 family therapies for adolescent anorexia nervosa: a randomized parallel trial. JAMA Psychiatry 2014;72(11): 1279–86.
55. Dalle Grave R, Calugi S, Doll H, et al. Enhanced cognitive behavioral therapy for adolescents with anorexia nervosa: an alternative to family therapy? Behav Res Ther 2013;51:R9–12.
56. Robin A, Siegal P, Moye A, et al. A controlled comparison of family versus individual therapy for adolescents with anorexia nervosa. J Am Acad Child Adolesc Psychiatry 1999;38(12):1482–9.
57. Lock J, Le Grange D, Agras WS, et al. A randomized clinical trial comparing family-based treatment to adolescent-focused individual therapy for adolescents with anorexia nervosa. Arch Gen Psychiatry 2010;67(10):1025–32.
58. Forsberg S, LoTempio E, Bryson S, et al. Therapeutic alliance in two treatments for adolescent anorexia nervosa. Int J Eat Disord 2013;46:34–8.
59. Walsh BT, Kaplan AS, Attia E, et al. Fluoxetine after weight restoration in anorexia nervosa: a randomized clinical trial. JAMA 2006;295:2605–12.
60. Hagman J, Gralla J, Sigel E, et al. A double-blind, placebo-controlled study of risperidone for the treatment of adolescents and young adults with anorexia nervosa: a pilot study. J Am Acad Child Adolesc Psychiatry 2011;50:915–24.
61. Davis H, Attia E. Pharmacology of eating disorders. Curr Opin Psychiatry 2017; 30(6):452–7.
62. Couturier J, Lock J. Review of medication use for children and adolescents with eating disorders. J Can Acad Child Adolesc Psychiatry 2007;16:173–6.
63. Doyle P, Le Grange D, Loeb K, et al. Early response to family-based treatment for adolescent anorexia nervosa. Int J Eat Disord 2010;43(7):659–62.

64. Fitzpatrick K, Darcy A, Le Grange D, et al. In vivo meal training for initial nonre-sponders. In: Loeb K, Le Grange D, Lock J, editors. Family therapy for adolescent eating and weight disorders: new applications. New York: Routledge; 2015. p. 45–58.
65. Byrne C, Accurso E, Arnow K, et al. An exploratory examination of patient and parental self-efficacy as predictors of weight gain in adolescents with anorexia nervosa. Int J Eat Disord 2015;48(7):883–8.
66. Sadeh-Sharvit S, Arnow K, Osipov L, et al. Are parental self-efficacy and family flexibility mediators of treatment for anorexia nervosa. Int J Eat Disord 2018; 51(3):275–80.
67. Roberts M, Tchanturia K, Stahl D, et al. A systematic review and meta-analysis of set-shifting ability in eating disorders. Psychol Med 2007;37:1075–84.
68. Tchanturia K, Davies H. Cognitive remediation. In: Grilo C, Mitchel J, editors. The treatment of eating disorder: clinical handbook. New York: Guilford Press; 2009. p. 130–50.
69. Eisler I, Dare C, Hodes M, et al. Family therapy for adolescent anorexia nervosa: the results of a controlled comparison of two family interventions. J Child Psychol Psychiatry 2000;41(6):727–36.
70. Le Grange D, Eisler I, Dare C, et al. Evaluation of family treatments in adolescent anorexia nervosa: a pilot study. Int J Eat Disord 1992;12(4):347–57.
71. Eisler I, Simic M, Hodsoll J, et al. A pragmatic randomised multi-centre trial of multifamily and single family therapy for adolescent anorexia nervosa. BMC Psychiatry 2016;16(1):422–35.
72. Dare C, Eisler I. A multi-family group day treatment programme for adolescent eating disorders. Eur Eat Disord Rev 2000;8:4–18.
73. Le Grange D, Lock J, Agras W, et al. Moderators and mediators of remission in family-based treatment and adolescent focused therapy for anorexia nervosa. Behav Res Ther 2012;50:85–92.

Update on Treatments for Adolescent Bulimia Nervosa

Sasha Gorrell, PhD[a], Daniel Le Grange, PhD[a,b],*

KEYWORDS

- Eating disorders • Bulimia nervosa • Family-based treatment

KEY POINTS

- A dearth of randomized controlled trials in adolescent bulimia nervosa (BN) has limited treatment advances.
- Family-based treatment is an evidence-based treatment for adolescent BN.
- Future research is needed to determine for whom, and under what conditions, certain types of family involvement might be most effective in the treatment of adolescent BN.

INTRODUCTION

First described by Gerald Russell nearly 40 years ago,[1] bulimia nervosa (BN) is an eating disorder (ED) broadly characterized by recurrent episodes of binge eating (ie, eating an objectively large quantity of food with an associated loss of control), followed by engagement in compensatory behaviors (eg, self-induced vomiting; misuse of laxatives, diuretics, or other medication; fasting; excessive exercise). These maladaptive compensatory behaviors are engaged to prevent or offset anticipated weight gain, and are concurrent with overvaluation of weight and shape.[2] The fifth edition of the *Diagnostic and Statistical Manual for Mental Disorders* (DSM-5) specifies that these episodes of binge eating and compensatory behavior must occur at a minimum frequency of once per week over the course of 3 months.[2]

To address these symptoms among adults with BN, a large number of randomized controlled trials (RCTs) testing psychotherapy, pharmacotherapy, or their combination, have demonstrated consistent support for the efficacy of cognitive behavioral therapy (CBT) as compared with other active treatments.[3,4] In addition, one study

Funded by: NIH. Grant number(s): T32 MH018261 (Pffifner)
Disclosure Statement: Dr S. Gorrell has no commercial relationships to disclose. Dr D. Le Grange receives royalties from Guilford Press and Routledge, and is co-director of the Training Institute for Child and Adolescent Eating Disorders, LLC.
[a] Department of Psychiatry, University of California, San Francisco, 401 Parnassus Avenue, San Francisco, CA 94143, USA; [b] The University of Chicago, Chicago, IL, USA
* Corresponding author. 401 Parnassus Avenue, San Francisco, CA 94143.
E-mail address: Daniel.LeGrange@ucsf.edu

found that interpersonal psychotherapy demonstrated parity with CBT in treating BN among adult samples, although with a slower course in reaching effectiveness.[5,6]

Turning to the examination of treatment efficacy among adolescents, in contrast with robust evidence from treatment studies among adults, research trials for BN in youth are vastly underrepresented.[7] To date, there has been 1 open medication trial, and 4 published RCTs comparing psychosocial treatments for adolescents, with substantial room for improvement in treatment outcomes (**Table 1**). The dearth of RCTs in this population is not an indication or reflection of low base rates of the disorder, as approximately 1% to 2% of adolescents meet full criteria for a diagnosis of BN, and an additional 2% to 3% may present with clinically meaningful subclinical BN.[8] Further, community studies evaluating disordered eating behavior found far greater prevalence of BN (14%–22%) when not adhering strictly to DSM-based criteria.[9,10] Of those afflicted, up to 40% may experience significant psychiatric comorbidity[11] or elevated suicidality.[12] In adolescence, prevalence estimates of BN are more than twice that of anorexia nervosa (AN).[10] Given evidence that medical hazards of BN are comparable with the more widely documented perils of AN,[13] effective treatment of BN in adolescents is essential.

TREATMENT
Psychopharmacological Treatment

Evidence-based pharmacologic treatment for children and adolescents with EDs generally, and in BN more specifically, is not yet possible because of the limited number of published studies. As a consequence, current clinical guidelines for treating BN in youth and adolescents do not include the use of psychopharmacology, other than to state that medication should not be offered as a sole treatment option.[14] However, the utility (or lack thereof) of pharmacotherapy in BN has been well established in adult populations, and in particular with selective serotonin reuptake inhibitors (SSRIs), such as fluoxetine.[15,16] In addition to several other trials, fluoxetine has been investigated for use among adults who have been categorized as "nonresponders" in the context of psychosocial treatments, with encouraging outcomes.[17] In adult studies, potential participants declined to participate in clinical medication trials citing concerns regarding potential side effects (eg, insomnia) or because of skepticism regarding the use of medication for a behavioral problem.[17] Further, although the use of fluoxetine has regulatory approval for treatment of BN in adults, for adolescents this only one open clinical trial was published investigating the feasibility, tolerability, and preliminary efficacy of fluoxetine in conjunction with psychotherapy over the course of 8 weeks.[18] In this study, 10 female adolescents (aged 12–18 years) with a DSM-IV diagnosis of BN or ED Not Otherwise Specified (EDNOS) received an adult dose of 60 mg of fluoxetine. Results indicated that the medication was well tolerated, and no participants discontinued the trial due to adverse effects. Findings indicated a significant reduction in binge eating and purging episodes over the course of the trial, at a weekly decrease of 67% and 56%, respectively.

Although it seems as if antidepressants are similarly useful and well tolerated for the treatment of adolescent BN as with adults, these findings have not yet been replicated nor have there been any placebo-controlled trials in adolescents with BN. Given evidence suggesting that the combination of antidepressant medication with psychotherapy leads to optimal treatment effects among some adults with BN,[19,20] it is surprising that both study and implementation of medication among adolescents with BN has been rather limited. Medication use for EDs has lagged behind other

Table 1
Randomized controlled trials of adolescent treatment of bulimia nervosa

Author, Year	Sample	Comparison Groups	Primary Outcomes	Main Findings
Schmidt et al,[26] 2007	Meet criteria for DSM-IV BN or EDNOS: $N = 85$; aged 13–20	Family therapy (FT) ($n = 41$); self-guided Cognitive Behavioral Therapy (CBT-GS) ($n = 44$) Dose: 6 mo, FT: 13 sessions with close others + 2 individual; CBT: 10 weekly sessions, 3 monthly follow-up + 2 optional with a close other	Abstinence from binge eating and vomiting following 6 mo of treatment, and at 6-mo follow-up	CBT-GS demonstrated significantly greater reductions in binge eating at EOT as compared with FT; differences were not retained at 6-mo follow-up. No differences between groups at EOT in purging behavior or attitudinal symptoms. Direct cost of care reduced in CBT-GS, but groups did not differ across other cost categories.
Le Grange et al,[25] 2007	Meet criteria for DSM-IV BN or partial BN[a]: $N = 80$; aged 12–19	Family-Based Treatment for BN (FBT-BN) ($n = 41$); Supportive Psychotherapy (SPT) ($n = 39$) Dose: 20 sessions over 6 mo	Abstinence from binge-and-purge episodes for 4 wk before assessment, per EDE; measured at EOT and 6-mo follow-up	FBT-BN had significantly higher rates of abstinence from binge eating and purging episodes than SPT at EOT (39% vs 18%); across both groups, rate of abstinence declined when assessed at 12-mo (29% and 10%, respectively).
Le Grange et al,[29] 2015	Meet criteria for DSM-IV BN or partial BN: $N = 130$; aged 12–18	FBT-BN ($n = 51$); CBT adapted for adolescents (CBT-A) ($n = 58$); SPT (not included in analyses) Dose: 18 sessions over 6 mo	Abstinence from binge-and-purge episodes for 4 wk before assessment, per EDE; measured at EOT, 6-mo and 12-mo follow-up	FBT-BN had significantly higher rates of abstinence from binge eating and purging episodes than CBT-A at EOT (39% vs 20%) and at 6-mo follow-up (44% vs 25%). Abstinence rates between groups did not differ at 12- month follow-up (49% vs 32%).
Stefini et al,[32] 2017	Meet criteria for DSM-IV BN or partial BN: $N = 81$; aged 14–20	Psychodynamic Therapy (PDT) ($n = 42$); CBT ($n = 39$) Dose: 60 sessions over 12 mo	Remission, defined as a lack of DSM-IV diagnosis for BN or partial BN at EOT and 12-mo follow-up	No significant differences in remission rates between groups at EOT or at 12-mo follow-up. Both groups demonstrated improvement on all secondary outcomes with improved rates of binge eating and purging in favor of CBT and for eating concern, in favor of PDT.

Abbreviations: BN, bulimia nervosa; DSM, *Diagnostic and Statistical Manual of Mental Disorders*; EDE, Eating Disorder Examination; EDNOS, eating disorder not otherwise specified; EOT, end of treatment.
[a] Partial BN = those who endorsed binge-and-purge episodes averaging once per week over 6 months.

psychiatric disorders, and currently, no medication has regulatory approval for use among those with AN, both factors that may contribute to the paucity of its study among adolescents with BN. In addition, given that increased risk of suicidality has been reported for SSRIs in younger populations,[21] as well as in adolescents with BN,[12] it is imperative that clinicians who do choose to prescribe these medications monitor patients closely and discuss these risks with patients and families. Overall, findings from the single study of pharmacotherapy for adolescent BN remain limited in their generalizability, and additional exploration of psychopharmacological interventions in adolescents with BN is warranted.

Psychological Treatment

Although prevalence estimates for adolescent BN consistently surpass those of adolescent AN,[10] there is a comparatively limited amount of research evaluating psychological treatment outcomes in this population.[22] Treatment for EDs in youth and adolescents over the past half-century principally supports family therapy,[14,23] and current published clinical guidelines recommend an ED-specific family therapy treatment for adolescents with BN.[14,24] Guidelines further specify, should a family therapy approach be unacceptable, contraindicated, or ineffective, individual ED-focused CBT should be considered.[14]

To date, 3 of 4 published RCTs have specifically evaluated the efficacy of family therapy or family-based treatment (FBT) for adolescent BN. Notably, these trials represent fewer than one-third of published RCTs examining psychotherapy treatment, and specifically FBT approaches, among adolescents with AN. The first 2 RCTs for adolescent BN compared a family approach with an individual psychotherapy.[25,26] In the first of these 2 studies, 85 adolescents with BN or EDNOS were randomized to family therapy or to CBT-guided self-care.[26] This particular family-based approach was an adaptation of family therapy for AN for use with individuals with BN. In this trial, CBT-guided self-care was undertaken by the adolescent and supported by a health care professional. Primary outcomes were abstinence from binge eating and vomiting following 6 months of treatment, and a follow-up at 6 months posttreatment; secondary outcomes included attitudinal bulimic symptoms, and treatment cost. Results indicated that adolescents receiving CBT-guided self-care had significant reductions in binge eating at 6 months, but these differences were not retained at follow-up. Further, there were no differences between groups at end of treatment (EOT) in purging behavior or attitudinal symptoms. Direct cost of care was reduced in CBT-guided self-care; these findings have clinical relevance, as CBT-guided self-care might be easily conducted in nonspecialty clinics. Despite this cost advantage to CBT-guided self-care, primary findings from this study indicate that CBT-guided self-care did not evidence statistical superiority in the main outcome criteria, as compared with a family therapy approach at EOT. Certainly, reductions in clinical symptoms are clinically meaningful, but sustained recovery in the context of BN treatment should ultimately include the aim of abstinence.

In the same year, a manualized approach to family treatment for BN (FBT-BN) was used in a study comparing this treatment with an individual supportive psychotherapy (SPT).[25] In this first trial of manualized FBT-BN, 80 participants (aged 12–19) with a DSM-IV diagnosis of BN or partial BN (ie, those who endorsed binge eating and purge episodes averaging once per week over 6 months), were randomized to 1 of these 2 treatments, each for 20 sessions over 6 months.[25] SPT is a nondirective treatment that does not include specific active therapeutic elements. FBT-BN is characterized by an agnostic stance toward the etiology and pathogenesis of the ED, along with the overarching tenet that parents are a key and influential resource in their child's recovery process. In initial stages of treatment, FBT-BN mobilizes parental resources in disrupting the cycle of ED behaviors. As behavioral symptom resolution is facilitated, and weight restoration is achieved (if applicable), less parental authority is typically required and parents may gradually restore autonomy over eating behavior to the adolescent (for the published treatment manual, see Ref.[27]). Results indicated that those receiving FBT-BN had significantly higher rates of abstinence from binge eating and purging episodes (39% vs 18%, $P = .049$) at EOT; across both groups, the rate of abstinence declined when assessed at 12-month follow-up (29% and 10%, respectively, $P = .05$), although the rate between the 2 groups remained statistically in favor of FBT-BN. Further, secondary outcome assessment revealed main effects in favor of FBT-BN on all measures of eating pathology, as measured by the Eating Disorder Examination (EDE).[28] As the first test of a manualized specialty treatment for BN in a sample of adolescents, this trial demonstrated the clinical and statistical superiority of FBT-BN as compared with nonspecialty treatment. Abstinence rates for BN behaviors were 40% for FBT-BN, similar to abstinence rates typically achieved in CBT for BN in adults. Nonetheless, this result indicates a need to find avenues to improve abstinence rates, a strong predictor of longer-term recovery.

In a more recent trial, FBT-BN was compared with a version of CBT that was adapted for adolescents with BN (CBT-A).[29] In this study, 109 adolescents (aged 12–18) with a DSM-IV diagnosis of BN or partial BN (as defined previously) were randomized to CBT-A or FBT-BN, each for 18 sessions over 6 months. CBT-A is an individual therapy that focuses on reducing dieting and on amending maladaptive behaviors and cognitions specifically related to shape and weight.[30] Adaptations to CBT unique to this patient population included exploration of developmental challenges, and collateral sessions with parents with a focus on psychoeducation of BN. FBT-BN was delivered with the approach described in the earlier study (see Ref.[25]). Results indicate that abstinence from binge eating and purging episodes for the 28 days before treatment conclusion was statistically superior for FBT-BN as compared with CBT-A (39.4% vs 19.7%, $P = .04$). At 6-month follow-up, abstinence rates for both groups continued to improve, but remained significantly elevated for FBT-BN (44% and 25.4%, respectively, $P = .03$); between-group abstinence rates did not differ statistically at 12-month follow-up. It should be pointed out that although there was not a statistical difference between the groups at 12-month follow-up, the study was not powered for the follow-up analysis.

In recent secondary analyses of this study sample, both CBT-A and FBT-BN showed comparable improvement in self-esteem and depression scores at EOT, and at extended follow-up.[31] Given the elevated frequency of comorbid psychopathology, and in particular depressive symptoms, associated with BN,[11] reduction in these symptoms is of considerable importance within the context of any treatment approach. Despite evidence that FBT-BN is more effective than CBT-A in achieving abstinence from binge eating and purging behaviors, some families may advocate for an individual therapy, with the commonly held assumption that such an approach would better help with depressive symptoms as well as BN symptoms. Findings from this most recent secondary analysis suggest that although not an explicit focus of treatment, mechanisms within FBT may indirectly impact depressive symptoms.[31] Further investigation of this mechanism is warranted, but current evidence may, in the meantime, help to guide clinicians and caretakers in selecting appropriate treatment options for adolescents with BN who present with lower self-esteem and elevated depressive symptoms.

Divergent from the previous work investigating FBT, the most recent trial of adolescent BN compared CBT with psychodynamic therapy (PDT).[32] Participants in this study were girls and young women (aged 14–20) with a DSM-IV diagnosis of BN or partial BN (ie, those who averaged binge eating and purging episodes less than twice per week in the previous 3 months). In alignment with standard treatment guidelines of clinical practice in Germany, both CBT and PDT took place over 1 year, and participants could receive up to 60 outpatient treatment sessions. CBT was based on a model of CBT for EDs,[33] and PDT was manualized specifically for young persons with BN. Both treatments share a symptom-focused approach, specific to BN, but with considerably divergent theoretic assumptions about the etiology and maintenance of the disorder. At the conclusion of treatment, there were no differences between groups on the primary outcome measure, that is, the number of individuals who no longer met diagnostic criteria for an ED (33.3% of those receiving CBT vs 30.2% receiving PDT). At 12-month follow-up, rates of remission improved slightly for CBT, albeit not significantly, whereas rates for PDT remained unchanged. The primary conclusion from this study suggests that parity in important indicators of recovery may be achieved with CBT and PDT approaches alike in adolescent BN. However, for many individuals within health care systems that do not subsidize extended methods of care, such as the United States, the number of sessions afforded to patients in this trial is not achievable. Future trials of abbreviated versions of these 2 treatment approaches may provide critical information about whether extended courses of intervention are necessary.

Taken together, 4 RCTs among adolescents are a fraction of the plethora of treatment studies conducted among adults with BN. It is possible that the dearth of trials among youth and adolescents with BN is due to evidence that, on average, the age of individuals who present for treatment with full or partial syndrome BN, are older than those presenting for treatment for AN.[22] Further, individuals with BN are often fully symptomatic while still within normal weight ranges for their age and height, further increasing the likelihood that adolescents may miss early detection of this disorder in primary care settings, where referrals are often made.[34] Despite these factors that have possibly impeded treatment advancement among adolescents with BN, these 4 completed RCTs provide provisional, yet robust support for the psychological treatment of adolescent BN. In particular, 3 trials have investigated a family-focused approach, 2 of which have evaluated a manualized FBT-BN as compared with another distinct and active individual treatment (SPT, and CBT-A, respectively). In each, FBT-BN has demonstrated statistically, as well as clinically, superior rates of abstinence from binge eating and purging at treatment conclusion. Across all 4 treatment studies, FBT-BN results in expedited behavior change and elevated sustained abstinence rates that may be maintained up to 12 months posttreatment.

In summary, it appears that similarly to adolescents with AN, clinically meaningful outcomes can be achieved with adolescents with BN when an approach that actively involves their families is used in the treatment process. As no treatment tested to date demonstrates statistically superior outcomes after 12 months, families who cannot for one reason or another participate in treatment, or who would prefer individual treatment, or when an adolescent is unwilling to involve caretakers, may find that CBT treatment is a beneficial alternative.

MEDIATORS AND MODERATORS OF TREATMENT OUTCOME

In an effort to improve manualized ED treatment for BN, some effort to identify potential moderators and/or mediators of outcome that may lead to a better understanding of *how* these treatments work, as well as for *whom* these treatments work, has been undertaken. Mediators identify mechanisms by way of which a particular treatment may achieve its affects, whereas moderators are baseline variables that specify for whom, and under what conditions a treatment works.[35] Within the context of RCTs that investigate treatment for adolescent BN, both mediators and moderators are critical to our ability to discern which aspects of treatment may bring about optimal therapeutic change.[36] In comparison with comparable treatment methods for adolescent AN, as a field, clinicians and researchers alike know considerably less about how or for whom existing treatments work. Although much of the extant research on mediators and moderators across EDs has focused on individuals older than 16 years,[37] a recent review has been conducted of research among adolescent populations, within which information specifically regarding BN remains limited (see Ref.[38]).

The first explicit examination of moderators of treatment outcome in adolescent BN comes from the initial study of 80 adolescents randomized to either FBT-BN or SPT.[25] First examining early predictors of outcome, a 85% reduction in binge eating and purging by session 6, whether FBT-BN or SPT, predicted remission at EOT and at 6-month follow-up.[39] However, based on these initial findings, it is not tenable to assume that an early reduction in either behavioral or attitudinal symptoms is critical in the success of treatment in adolescent BN. Turning to moderators, participants with less severe ED psychopathology (lower EDE Global scores), who received FBT-BN, were more likely to meet criteria for partial remission (ie, no longer meeting diagnosis or study entry criteria) at 6-month follow-up than those who received SPT.[40] In terms of mediators, early symptom remission was impactful on outcomes.[41] FBT-BN was particularly efficacious in bringing about remission at EOT (ie, absence of binge eating and purging in the prior 4 weeks) by way of early (midtreatment/session 10) reductions in ED pathology (ie, change in EDE-Questionnaire [EDE-Q] subscales).[42] All EDE-Q subscales were significant mediators of treatment outcome, suggesting that FBT-BN exerts its effects by changing disordered thinking relatively early on in treatment. The mechanism of change, or how FBT-BN brings about this change, has not been the subject of systematic inquiry.

In only the second, and to date largest, study to explore moderators of treatment outcome, Le Grange and colleagues[29] examined 29 baseline variables within an RCT of 109 adolescents randomized to either CBT-A or FBT-AN.[29] Among the many variables considered, only the Family Environment Scale (FES)[43] assessment of conflict was identified as a treatment effect moderator. Participants with a lower FES conflict score responded better to FBT-BN as compared with CBT-A.

Considered together, these preliminary studies of potential moderators and mediators of treatment outcome for adolescent BN suggest that individuals with more severe symptom presentation at the start of treatment may fair better with FBT-BN, rather than SPT.[40] Further, although family structure itself may not impact treatment outcome, adolescents exposed to less parental conflict may also fair better in FBT-BN treatment, as compared with CBT-A.[29] In general, for those who demonstrate early indication of nonresponse to treatment, identification of the potential moderators or mediators that may be driving nonresponse is critical. Although these preliminary findings of potential moderators and mediators provide useful information along with suggested clinical guidelines, future studies with sufficient power to examine either mediators or moderators as a priori hypotheses would aid in improved understanding of how FBT-BN exerts its influence. Continued examination of factors that increase adaptive treatment response may ultimately help to guide future treatment refinement and development.

FUTURE DIRECTIONS

A paucity of RCTs in adolescent BN has limited treatment advances, despite a widely acknowledged notion that treatments for adolescents with eating disorders must improve.[44] Notably, the 2 trials described previously that compare the efficacy of a manualized FBT-BN approach with another distinct and active individual psychotherapy (SPT and CBT-A, respectively) provide support for the use of FBT as a first-line treatment for adolescents with a diagnosis of BN. However, the dearth of current evidence in treatment trials for this patient population falls demonstrably short of that among both adult samples with BN, as well as in other adolescent ED samples (eg, AN).

Current research in AN, supports early weight gain as an important predictor of improved treatment outcome.[45] By comparison, we have yet to consistently establish that decreased ED pathology, or even potentially early cessation of binge eating and purging may lead to similar positive treatment outcomes in adolescent BN. In addition, although decreased family conflict[29] and baseline ED pathology[40] are potential moderators of FBT-BN treatment, future work should examine other moderators that have been identified in AN, including parental self-efficacy[46] and parental criticism.[47] To improve outcomes, it is of critical importance to study how family-based interventions in adolescent BN achieve symptom remission, or lead to other positive treatment outcomes. Early indications that decreased ED pathology may mediate differences in abstinence from binge eating and purging behavior following treatment are encouraging.[41]

In addition to the examination of for *whom* FBT-BN is beneficial, or *how* FBT-BN elicits symptom change, it is critical that future studies improve adolescent BN treatment outcomes by exploring different formats of this treatment. For example, based on promising results demonstrated within samples of youth with AN,[48,49] FBT may be expanded to a multifamily or intensive family treatment format (IFT). In IFT, families participate in a 5-day, 8 hours per day, treatment week; this efficient format may be particularly helpful for families who cannot regularly access specialty ED care, and may also serve as an option for particularly severe cases.[50] Integrated within an IFT approach, a multiple-family format is predicated on the supposition that when families are brought together in groups, family resources and support for one another are amplified, which may then lead to improved outcomes.[51] Another necessary consideration in treatment format derives from the high level of psychiatric comorbidity associated with BN.[11] This clinical feature increases the likelihood that adolescents may present for treatment of another disorder (eg, mood, anxiety, or substance use disorder) while also reporting symptoms of binge eating and purging.[52] Therefore, it is critical that future studies investigate whether consecutive or concurrent treatment approaches for comorbid diagnoses are most appropriate or effective for this subset of this patient population.

One of the most important challenges in advancing empirically based treatment for adolescent BN, in addition to improving efficacy, is increasing its availability to more individuals and families who could benefit from the current manualized FBT-BN approach. Access to specialty providers for ED treatment is a particular challenge outside of urban environs, with a limited number of trained providers outside the sites where FBT was developed.[53] Increasing access to FBT training for clinicians through Web-based education and supervision is a key area of future development. Although preliminary effectiveness for the delivery of FBT via Telehealth has been established for adolescent AN,[54,55] this platform for the delivery of FBT-BN remains unexplored. Therefore, further examination of this dissemination method is warranted both across a larger trial, and specifically among adolescents with BN.

SUMMARY

Currently, there are few systematic studies of treatment of BN in adolescents. Although RCTs of FBT-BN for adolescents have demonstrated evidence to support the focused involvement of parents in treatment, there remains a need for improved and sustainable outcomes in reducing binge eating and purging symptoms over time. In instances in which parents are unable or perhaps unwilling to participate in treatment, there is evidence that individual ED-specific CBT approaches are helpful for some adolescents. Further investigation of treatment approaches for adolescents with BN, psychosocial as well as pharmacologic, will counteract the current paucity of research evidence, and contribute to treatment advancement in this vulnerable population.

REFERENCES

1. Russell G. Bulimia nervosa: an ominous variant of anorexia nervosa. Psychol Med 1979;9(3):429–48.
2. American Psychiatric Association. Diagnostic and statistical manual of mental disorders. 5th edition. Washington, DC: APA; 2013.
3. Shapiro JR, Berkman ND, Brownley KA, et al. Bulimia nervosa treatment: a systematic review of randomized controlled trials. Int J Eat Disord 2007;40(4): 321–36.
4. Poulsen S, Lunn S, Daniel SI, et al. A randomized controlled trial of psychoanalytic psychotherapy or cognitive-behavioral therapy for bulimia nervosa. Focus 2014;12(4):450–8.
5. Agras WS, Walsh T, Fairburn CG, et al. A multicenter comparison of cognitive-behavioral therapy and interpersonal psychotherapy for bulimia nervosa. Arch Gen Psychiatry 2000;57(5):459–66.
6. Fairburn CG, Bailey-Straebler S, Basden S, et al. A transdiagnostic comparison of enhanced cognitive behaviour therapy (CBT-E) and interpersonal psychotherapy in the treatment of eating disorders. Behav Res Ther 2015;70:64–71.
7. Hail L, Le Grange D. Bulimia nervosa in adolescents: prevalence and treatment challenges. Adolesc Health Med Ther 2018;9:11.
8. Smink FRE, van Hoeken D, Hoek HW. Epidemiology of eating disorders: incidence, prevalence and mortality rates. Curr Psychiatry Rep 2012;14:406–14.
9. Jones JM, Bennett S, Olmsted MP, et al. Disordered eating attitudes and behaviours in teenaged girls: a school-based study. CMAJ 2001;165(5):547–52.
10. Swanson SA, Crow S, Le Grange D, et al. Prevalence and correlates of eating disorders in adolescents: results from the national comorbidity survey replication adolescent supplement. Arch Gen Psychiatry 2011;68(7):714–23.
11. Thompson-Brenner H, Westen D. A naturalistic study of psychotherapy for bulimia nervosa, part 1: comorbidity and therapeutic outcome. J Nerv Ment Dis 2005;193:573–84.
12. Crow SJ, Swanson SA, Le Grange D, et al. Suicidal behavior in adolescents and adults with bulimia nervosa. Compr Psychiatry 2014;55(7):1534–9.
13. Crow S, Peterson C, Swanson S, et al. Increased mortality in bulimia nervosa and other eating disorders. Am J Psychiatry 2009;166:1342–6.
14. National Institute for Health and Care Excellence. Eating disorders: recognition and treatment (NICE guideline NH69). 2017. Available at: https://www.nice.org.uk/guidance/ng69. Accessed June 17, 2019.
15. Davis H, Attia E. Pharmacotherapy of eating disorders. Curr Opin Psychiatry 2017;30(6):452–7.
16. Walsh BT, Kaplan AS, Attia E, et al. Fluoxetine after weight restoration in anorexia nervosa: a randomized controlled trial. JAMA 2006;295(22):2605–12.

17. Walsh BT, Agras WS, Devlin MJ, et al. Fluoxetine for bulimia nervosa following poor response to psychotherapy. Am J Psychiatry 2000;157(8):1332–4.
18. Kotler L, Devlin MJ, Davies M, et al. An open trial of fluoxetine for adolescents with bulimia nervosa. J Child Adolesc Psychopharmacol 2003;13(3):329–35.
19. Flament MF, Bissada H, Spettigue W. Evidence-based pharmacotherapy of eating disorders. Int J Neuropsychopharmacol 2012;15(2):189–207.
20. Walsh BT, Wilson GT, Loeb KL, et al. Medication and psychotherapy in the treatment of bulimia nervosa. Am J Psychiatry 1997;154(4):523–31.
21. Morrison J, Schwartz TL. Adolescent angst or true intent? Suicidal behavior, risk, and neurobiological mechanisms in depressed children and teenagers taking antidepressants. Int J Emerg Ment Health 2014;16(1):247–50.
22. Le Grange D, Loeb KL, Van Orman S, et al. Bulimia nervosa in adolescents: a disorder in evolution? Arch Pediatr Adolesc Med 2004;158(5):478–82.
23. Lock J, Le Grange D. Family-based treatment: where are we and where should we be going to improve recovery in child and adolescent eating disorders. Int J Eat Disord 2019;52(4):481–7.
24. Hilbert A, Hoek HW, Schmidt R. Evidence-based clinical guidelines for eating disorders: international comparison. Curr Opin Psychiatry 2017;30(6):423.
25. Le Grange D, Crosby RD, Rathouz PJ, et al. A randomized controlled comparison of family-based treatment and supportive psychotherapy for adolescent bulimia nervosa. Arch Gen Psychiatry 2007;64(9):1049–56.
26. Schmidt U, Lee S, Beecham J, et al. A randomized controlled trial of family therapy and cognitive behavior therapy guided self-care for adolescents with bulimia nervosa and related disorders. Am J Psychiatry 2007;164(4):591–8.
27. Le Grange D, Lock J. Treating bulimia in adolescents: a family-based approach. New York: Guilford Press; 2007.
28. Fairburn CG, Cooper I. The eating disorder examination. In: Fairburn CG, Wilson GT, editors. Binge eating: nature, assessment, and treatment. 12th edition. New York: Guilford Press; 1993.
29. Le Grange D, Lock J, Agras WS, et al. Randomized clinical trial of family-based treatment and cognitive-behavioral therapy for adolescent bulimia nervosa. J Am Acad Child Adolesc Psychiatry 2015;54(11):886–94.
30. Lock J. Adjusting cognitive behavior therapy for adolescents with bulimia nervosa: results of case series. Am J Psychother 2005;59(3):267–81.
31. Valenzuela F, Lock J, Le Grange D, et al. Comorbid depressive symptoms and self-esteem improve after either cognitive-behavioral therapy or family-based treatment for adolescent bulimia nervosa. Eur Eat Disord Rev 2018;26:253–8.
32. Stefini A, Salzer S, Reich G, et al. Cognitive-behavioral and psychodynamic therapy in female adolescents with bulimia nervosa: a randomized controlled trial. J Am Acad Child Adolesc Psychiatry 2017;56(4):329–35.
33. Fairburn CG, Cooper Z, Shafran R. Enhanced cognitive behavior therapy for eating disorders (CBT-E): an overview. In: Fairburn CG, editor. Cognitive behavior therapy and eating disorders. New York: Guilford Press; 2008. p. 23–34.
34. Walsh JM, Wheat ME, Freund K. Detection, evaluation, and treatment of eating disorders. J Gen Intern Med 2000;15(8):577–90.
35. Baron RM, Kenny DA. The moderator-mediator variable distinction in social psychological research: conceptual, strategic, and statistical considerations. J Pers Soc Psychol 1986;51:1173–82.
36. Kraemer HC, Wilson GT, Fairburn CG, et al. Mediators and moderators of treatment effects in randomized clinical trials. Arch Gen Psychiatry 2002;59(10):877–83.

37. Linardon J, de la Piedad Garcia X, Brennan L. Predictors, moderators, and me-diators of treatment outcome following manualised cognitive-behavioural therapy for eating disorders: a systematic review. Eur Eat Disord Rev 2017;25(1):3–12.
38. Murray S, Loeb K, Le Grange D. Mediators and moderators of treatment out-comes in adolescent eating disorders. In: Maric M, Prins P, Ollendick T, editors. Mediators and moderators of youth treatment outcome. New York: Oxford Univer-sity Press; 2015. p. 210–29.
39. Le Grange D, Doyle P, Crosby R, et al. Early response to treatment in adolescent bulimia nervosa. Int J Eat Disord 2008;41:755–7.
40. Le Grange D, Crosby RD, Lock J. Predictors and moderators of outcome in family-based treatment for adolescent bulimia nervosa. J Am Acad Child Adolesc Psychiatry 2008;47(4):464–70.
41. Lock J, Le Grange D, Crosby R. Exploring possible mechanisms of change in fam-ily-based treatment for adolescent bulimia nervosa. J Fam Ther 2008;30(3):260–71.
42. Fairburn CG, Beglin SJ. Assessment of eating disorders: interview or self-report questionnaire? Int J Eat Disord 1994;16(4):363–70.
43. Moos R, Moos B. Family environment scale manual. 3rd edition. Palo Alto (CA): Consulting Psychologists Press; 1994.
44. Lock J. An update on evidence-based psychological treatments for eating disor-ders in children and adolescents. J Clin Child Adolesc Psychol 2015;12:1–15.
45. Le Grange D, Accurso EC, Lock J, et al. Early weight gain predicts outcome in two treatments for adolescent anorexia nervosa. Int J Eat Disord 2014;47(2):124–9.
46. Byrne CE, Accurso EC, Arnow KD, et al. An exploratory examination of patient and parental self-efficacy as predictors of weight gain in adolescents with anorexia nervosa. Int J Eat Disord 2015;48(7):883–8.
47. Le Grange D, Hughes EK, Court A, et al. Randomized clinical trial of parent-focused treatment and family-based treatment for adolescent anorexia nervosa. J Am Acad Child Adolesc Psychiatry 2016;55:683–92.
48. Marzola E, Knatz S, Murray SB, et al. Short-term intensive family therapy for adolescent eating disorders: 30-month outcome. Eur Eat Disord Rev 2015; 23(3):210–8.
49. Rockwell RE, Boutelle K, Trunko ME, et al. An innovative short-term, intensive, family-based treatment for adolescent anorexia nervosa: case series. Eur Eat Dis-ord Rev 2011;19(4):362–7.
50. Knatz S, Kaye W, Marzola E, et al. A brief, intensive application of family based treatment for eating disorders. In: Loeb KL, Le Grange D, Lock J, editors. Family therapy for adolescent eating and weight disorders: new applications. New York: Routledge/Taylor and Francis Group; 2015. p. 72–91.
51. Eisler I, Simic M, Hodsoll J, et al. A pragmatic randomised multi-centre trial of multifamily and single family therapy for adolescent anorexia nervosa. BMC Psy-chiatry 2016;16(1):422.
52. Le Grange D, Schmidt U. The treatment of adolescents with bulimia nervosa. J Ment Health 2005;14(6):587–97.
53. Murray SB, Le Grange D. Family therapy for adolescent eating disorders: an up-date. Curr Psychiatry Rep 2014;16(5):447.
54. Anderson KE, Byrne C, Goodyear A, et al. Telemedicine of family-based treat-ment for adolescent anorexia nervosa: a protocol of a treatment development study. J Eat Disord 2015;3(1):25.
55. Anderson KE, Byrne CE, Crosby RD, et al. Utilizing Telehealth to deliver family-based treatment for adolescent anorexia nervosa. Int J Eat Disord 2017;50(10): 1235–8.

Binge Eating Disorder in Children and Adolescents

Cara Bohon, PhD

KEYWORDS

- Binge eating disorder • Binge eating • Obesity • Children • Adolescents
- Loss-of-control eating

KEY POINTS

- Binge eating disorder is prevalent in children and adolescents, often showing onset during adolescence.
- Current evidence-based treatments exist for adults with binge eating disorder, but research in children and adolescents is needed.
- In diagnosing binge eating in children, loss of control over eating may be more important than an objectively large amount of food.
- Despite greater incidence of binge eating disorder in male patients than other eating disorders, there is still a higher incidence of binge eating disorder in female patients.

INTRODUCTION

Binge eating is defined as the consumption of an objectively large amount of food (larger than what most people would consume under similar circumstances) coupled with a sense of loss of control (LOC) over the eating.[1] Binge eating disorder (BED) is characterized by recurrent episodes of binge eating, in addition to associated features such as distress about the eating, secrecy of eating, or eating in the absence of hunger.[1] Binge eating was first described by Albert Stunkard[2] in the 1950s but was not integrated into clinical diagnoses until the 1980 publication of the *Diagnostic and Statistical Manual of Mental Disorders* (DSM), 3rd edition, with the addition of bulimia, which was later renamed bulimia nervosa. In subsequent DSM editions, the understanding of binge eating increased, leading to the inclusion of BED as a formal diagnosis in the DSM-5 in 2013.

BED is commonly associated with obesity because the diagnosis is distinguished from bulimia nervosa by the absence of compensatory behaviors to eliminate calories consumed. Thus, recent studies of BED in children and adolescents have

Disclosure Statement: The author has no relationships to disclose.
Department of Psychiatry and Behavioral Sciences, Stanford University School of Medicine, 401 Quarry Road, Stanford, CA 94305-5719, USA
E-mail address: cbohon@stanford.edu

used samples of children who were overweight or obese. Initial research on binge eating, however, was in the context of bulimia nervosa in normal-weight adolescents. A historical review of this research has been conducted.[3] The association between binge eating and obesity leads to direct physical health consequences, and there are also associated psychological consequences, such as greater rates of depression.[4,5]

DIAGNOSIS

As noted, the DSM-5 defines BED as the recurrence of binge eating episodes characterized by

- The consumption of a large amount of food
- LOC over eating (**Table 1**).

These episodes must occur at least once per week on average over the prior 3 months. A diagnosis of other specified feeding and eating disorder: BED of low frequency or duration would be given to someone with less frequent or enduring binge episodes. In addition to the binge episodes, individuals meeting BED criteria must endorse at least 3 of the following features:

- Eating much more rapidly than normal
- Eating until feeling uncomfortably full
- Eating large amounts of food when not physical hungry
- Eating alone due to embarrassment about how much one is eating
- Feeling disgusted with oneself, depressed, or very guilty after overeating.

Finally, the diagnosis requires distress regarding binge eating and the absence of compensatory behaviors (eg, purging).

The diagnosis of binge episodes in children and adolescents can be challenging for several reasons. First, the definition of an objectively large amount of food during development can be difficult and uncertain.[6,7] Indeed, a child's caloric intake may vary due to growth spurts and changes in activity.[8] Furthermore, report of food intake, as well as the ability to articulate LOC, can be challenging in children and adolescents. For this reason, clinician-expert interviews are necessary rather than reliance on self-report to better characterize an eating episode as a binge.[9] Even with interviews, clinicians still rely on self-reported food intake, which is poorly related to actual objectively measured intake.[10] Verbal descriptions of portion and/or pictures of portions of food may aid in the assessment.[11]

Second, the criterion of LOC may be difficult for children and adolescents to understand. Tanofsky-Kraff and colleagues[7] have used terms such as numbing or zoning out to help children conceptualize LOC. Although challenging to assess, the inclusion of LOC in the measurement of binge eating is vital because it is associated with more psychosocial impairment than overeating alone.[6] Marcus and Kalarchian[12] proposed alternative BED criteria for children that highlight the

Table 1 Criteria for binge eating episode		
	Large Amount of Food	**Not Large Amount of Food**
LOC over eating	Objective binge episode	Subjective binge episode
No LOC	Overeating	Normal eating

LOC feature and eliminate the objectively large amount of food. Their criteria include

- Recurrent episodes of binge eating, defined by both of the following
  - Food seeking in the absence of hunger (eg, after a full meal)
  - A sense of lack of control over eating (eg, endorse that "When I start to eat, I just can't stop")
- Binge episodes are associated with 1 or more of the following
  - Food seeking in response to negative affect (eg, sadness, boredom, restlessness)
  - Food seeking as a reward
  - Sneaking or hiding food
- Symptoms persist over a period of 3 months
- Eating is not associated with the regular use of inappropriate compensatory behaviors (eg, purging, fasting, excessive exercise) and does not occur exclusively during the course of anorexia nervosa or bulimia nervosa.

These criteria were not officially adopted into the DSM-5, nor have they received much direct investigation through research. However, they are included here to highlight the uncertainty about whether the current criteria can be applied to children and adolescents without adaptation.

PREVALENCE, RISK, AND CONSEQUENCES

Several studies have attempted to estimate prevalence, incidence, and sex differences in BED in adolescents and children. There is a range of numbers for these values, in part due to differences in measurement or assessment tools used for BED, in particular self-report survey versus diagnostic interviews. Most studies reveal prevalence rates between 1% and 3%, with about twice as many girls reporting binge eating compared with boys.[13]

Risks for the development of BED are not definitively known, particularly for childhood binge eating. However, a study of very young children followed from birth to age 5 years was able to identify that maternal eating disinhibition, hunger, body dissatisfaction, body mass index (BMI), and a history of being overweight predicted secretive eating by age 5 years in the child.[14] Although secretive eating is not equivalent to binge eating, a feature of binge eating for BED diagnosis is eating alone due to embarrassment, which may be related. Other prospective studies of risk factors for BED have identified dieting and negative affect as consistent risk factors for binge eating.[15–18] Overvaluation of weight predicted weekly binge eating in a sample of overweight adolescent girls.[5] Eating in the absence of hunger and LOC eating in childhood predicted BED and binge eating behavior in adolescence.[19,20] Among children who displayed eating in the absence of hunger at age 7 years, BMI, anxiety, depression, dietary restraint, emotional disinhibition, and body dissatisfaction predicted binge eating at age 15 years.[19]

Age of onset for BED seems to be during late adolescence, although estimates range into early adulthood.[12,21] One study of treatment-seeking children and adolescents with obesity found greater odds of binge eating in white compared with African American patients,[4] although studies of adults have found similar rates of binge eating in black and white women.[22]

Youth with binge eating have higher adiposity, waist circumference, depressive symptoms, and disordered eating.[4] Children with persistent LOC eating older than 4 to 5 years showed greater depressive symptoms and disordered eating attitudes than those without LOC eating.[20] Among adolescent girls who were overweight and were engaging in weekly binge eating, those who overvalued weight reported greater depressive symptoms.[5]

TREATMENT

Treatment of BED in children and adolescents has not been adequately studied. To date, only a handful of studies have investigated such treatments in randomized controlled trials. Treatments for adult BED with current evidence in adults include guided self-help cognitive behavioral therapy (CBT) and interpersonal psychotherapy (IPT),[23] as well as dialectical behavior therapy (DBT).[24] CBT-based treatments focus on regulating eating patterns and addressing eating-related thoughts that contribute to symptoms. IPT aims to resolve interpersonal difficulties that are thought to maintain binge eating. DBT involves identifying emotion-related triggers to binge eating and teaching strategies to manage and tolerate those emotions without engaging in binge eating.

One study investigated the use of a 16-week CBT self-help online intervention for high school students who were greater than or equal to 85th percentile in BMI and engaging in binge eating or overeating at least once per week in the prior 3 months. It found that it reduced BMI z-scores and objective and subjective binge episodes, as well as reduced weight and shape concerns, compared with a waitlist control group.[25] Adolescents with more frequent objective overeating or binge eating at baseline had greater reductions in BMI at follow-up.[25] Another study conducted an 8-session CBT group-based intervention for adolescent girls with recurrent binge eating and found greater reductions in binge eating in the CBT group compared with treatment as usual.[26] A third trial investigated the use of a 12-session IPT group compared with a health education group in small sample of 12 to 17 year old girls. Of those with baseline LOC eating (n = 20), girls in the IPT group had greater reductions in LOC than those in the health education group. This finding was replicated in a larger sample with effects on LOC eating, as well as binge eating.[27] A case report of DBT in an adolescent patient suggested it could be adapted for use in this younger age group to treat BED, with the addition of family sessions.[28] Another study examined DBT-informed treatment of treating binge eating in adolescent girls with both DBT and a behavioral weight loss treatment showing reductions in eating disorder symptoms.[29]

Other studies assessing reductions in binge eating in response to treatment in youth have investigated the behavior in the context of weight loss treatments. One study found that binge eating was reduced after a 16-week CBT-based weight loss program.[30] The treatments included CBT components of behavior change, such as self-monitoring, problem-solving, motivation, and relapse prevention, as well as either a peer-enhanced adventure treatment or supervised aerobic exercise components.[30] Change in binge eating over the course of treatment was also associated with change in physical appearance self-concept, global self-concept, and physical self-worth.[30] Another study of behavioral and pharmacologic weight loss programs found that binge eating decreased over time with treatment and that baseline binge eating did not affect weight loss over the course of treatment.[31]

Given that family-based treatment (FBT) for anorexia nervosa and bulimia nervosa currently show some of the highest rates of remission for adolescents with those eating disorders,[32,33] it is likely that a family component or focus in the treatment of BED in children and adolescents would improve outcomes. Indeed, a trial of CBT for BED in adolescents ages 12 to 20 years that includes parent education is underway,[34] although results are not yet published. Even parent education, however, may not be sufficient because children's inhibitory control, which may be particularly relevant for an impulse control behavior such as binge eating, may still be developing naturally throughout adolescence.[35] FBT of BED would directly involve the family, particularly the parents, in helping the child or adolescent change behavior. Given the efficacy of FBT for bulimia nervosa, which also is characterized by recurrent binge eating, it is worth pursuing trials of this treatment of BED in this age group.

SUMMARY

BED is prevalent in children and adolescents and is associated with both physical and psychological impairments. Importantly, there is some controversy about whether the diagnosis should be modified for children, specifically focusing on LOC as the primary feature related to pathologic factors rather than the quantity of food consumed during an eating episode. Because many studies note late adolescence as the peak age of onset for BED, research on younger children and adolescents is particularly lacking. However, given that prevalence among younger samples is still high and the presence of any binge eating behavior is even greater,[13] it is vital that more resources be directed toward improving the identification, assessment, and treatment of BED in youth. A recent review confirmed this need, showing evidence that adolescents with BED are at increased risk of developing obesity, substance use, suicidality, and other psychological problems.[9]

Of note, although evidence suggests BED is more common in girls than boys, BED has the highest prevalence of any eating disorder in male patients. Despite this, most studies of treatments in adolescents have been conducted in female samples. Thus, there is a great need for studies examining treatments of BED in male adolescents. To date, there is a lack of strong evidence-based treatments, even for female adolescents, although preliminary evidence suggests that IPT, CBT, and DBT may show some efficacy. Internet or application-based interventions may be particularly fruitful given preliminary evidence supporting the use of an online intervention for binge eating in adolescents,[25] as well as findings that some adolescents may find online treatments more acceptable than in-person treatments.[36]

ACKNOWLEDGMENTS

The author is supported by grant from the National Institute of Mental Health (K23MH106794).

REFERENCES

1. American Psychiatric Association. Diagnostic and statistical manual of mental disorders, fifth edition (DSM-I5). Washington, DC: American Psychiatric Association; 2013.

2. Stunkard AJ. Eating patterns and obesity. Psychiatr Q 1959;33:284–95.

3. Chao A. Binge eating in obese adolescents: an evolutionary concept analysis. Nurs Forum (Auckl) 2014;49(3):189–99.

4. Elliott CA, Tanofsky-Kraff M, Mirza NM. Parent report of binge eating in Hispanic, African American and Caucasian youth. Eat Behav 2013;14(1):1–6.

5. Sonneville KR, Grilo CM, Richmond TK, et al. Prospective association between overvaluation of weight and binge eating among overweight adolescent girls. J Adolesc Health 2015;56(1):25–9.

6. Tanofsky-Kraff M, Goossens L, Eddy KT, et al. A multisite investigation of binge eating behaviors in children and adolescents. J Consult Clin Psychol 2007; 75(6):901–13.

7. Tanofsky-Kraff M, Yanovski SZ, Wilfley DE, et al. Eating-disordered behaviors, body fat, and psychopathology in overweight and normal-weight children. J Consult Clin Psychol 2004;72(1):53–61.

8. Institute of Medicine. Dietary reference intakes for energy, carbohydrate, fiber, fat, fatty acids, cholesterol, protein, and amino acids. Washington, DC: The National Acadmies Press; 2002.

9. Marzilli E, Cerniglia L, Cimino S. A narrative review of binge eating disorder in adolescence: prevalence, impact, and psychological treatment strategies. Adolesc Health Med Ther 2018;9:17–30.

10. Hill RJ, Davies PS. The validity of self-reported energy intake as determined using the doubly labelled water technique. Br J Nutr 2001;85(4):415–30.

11. Tanofsky-Kraff M, Yanovski SZ, Schvey NA, et al. A prospective study of loss of control eating for body weight gain in children at high risk for adult obesity. Int J Eat Disord 2009;42(1):26–30.

12. Marcus MD, Kalarchian MA. Binge eating in children and adolescents. Int J Eat Disord 2003;34(S1):S47–57.

13. Smink FRE, van Hoeken D, Oldehinkel AJ, et al. Prevalence and severity of DSM-5 eating disorders in a community cohort of adolescents. Int J Eat Disord 2014; 47(6):610–9.

14. Stice E, Agras WS, Hammer LD. Risk factors for the emergence of childhood eating disturbances: a five-year prospective study. Int J Eat Disord 1999;25(4): 375–87.

15. Johnson JG, Cohen P, Kotler L, et al. Psychiatric disorders associated with risk for the development of eating disorders during adolescence and early adulthood. J Consult Clin Psychol 2002;70(5):1119–28.

16. Stice E, Killen JD, Hayward C, et al. Age of onset for binge eating and purging during late adolescence: a 4-year survival analysis. J Abnorm Psychol 1998; 107(4):671–5.

17. Stice E, Gau JM, Rohde P, et al. Risk factors that predict future onset of each DSM-5 eating disorder: predictive specificity in high-risk adolescent females. J Abnorm Psychol 2017;126(1):38–51.

18. Stice E, Presnell K, Spangler D. Risk factors for binge eating onset in adolescent girls: a 2-year prospective investigation. Health Psychol 2002;21(2):131–8.

19. Balantekin KN, Birch LL, Savage JS. Eating in the absence of hunger during childhood predicts self-reported binge eating in adolescence. Eat Behav 2017; 24:7–10.

20. Tanofsky-Kraff M, Shomaker LB, Olsen C, et al. A prospective study of pediatric loss of control eating and psychological outcomes. J Abnorm Psychol 2011; 120(1):108–18.

21. Mustelin L, Raevuori A, Hoek HW, et al. Incidence and weight trajectories of binge eating disorder among young women in the community. Int J Eat Disord 2015; 48(8):1106–12.

22. Striegel-Moore RH, Wilfley DE, Pike KM, et al. Recurrent binge eating in black American women. Arch Fam Med 2000;9(1):83–7.

23. Wilson GT, Wilfley DE, Agras WS, et al. Psychological treatments of binge eating disorder. Arch Gen Psychiatry 2010;67(1):94–101.

24. Safer DL, Robinson AH, Jo B. Outcome from a randomized controlled trial of group therapy for binge eating disorder: comparing dialectical behavior therapy

adapted for binge eating to an active comparison group therapy. Behav Ther 2010;41(1):106–20.

25. Jones M, Luce KH, Osborne MI, et al. Randomized, controlled trial of an internet-facilitated intervention for reducing binge eating and overweight in adolescents. Pediatrics 2008;121(3):453–62.

26. DeBar LL, Wilson GT, Yarborough BJ, et al. Cognitive behavioral treatment for recurrent binge eating in adolescent girls: a pilot trial. Cogn Behav Pract 2013; 20(2):147–61.

27. Tanofsky-Kraff M, Shomaker LB, Wilfley DE, et al. Targeted prevention of excess weight gain and eating disorders in high-risk adolescent girls: a randomized controlled trial. Am J Clin Nutr 2014;100(4):1010–8.

28. Safer DL, Couturier JL, Lock J. Dialectical behavior therapy modified for adolescent binge eating disorder: a case report. Cogn Behav Pract 2007;14(2):157–67.

29. Mazzeo SE, Lydecker J, Harney M, et al. Development and preliminary effectiveness of an innovative treatment for binge eating in racially diverse adolescent girls. Eat Behav 2016;22:199–205.

30. Mehlenbeck RS, Jelalian E, Lloyd-Richardson EE, et al. Effects of behavioral weight control intervention on binge eating symptoms among overweight Adolescents. Psychol Sch 2009;46(8):776–86.

31. Bishop-Gilyard CT, Berkowitz RI, Wadden TA, et al. Weight reduction in obese adolescents with and without binge eating. Obesity (Silver Spring) 2011;19(5): 982–7.

32. Le Grange D, Lock J, Agras WS, et al. Randomized clinical trial of family-based treatment and cognitive-behavioral therapy for adolescent bulimia nervosa. J Am Acad Child Adolesc Psychiatry 2015;54(11):886–94.e2.

33. Lock J, Le Grange D. Family-based treatment: where are we and where should we be going to improve recovery in child and adolescent eating disorders. Int J Eat Disord 2018. https://doi.org/10.1002/eat.22980.

34. Hilbert A. Cognitive-behavioral therapy for binge eating disorder in adolescents: study protocol for a randomized controlled trial. Trials 2013;14:312.

35. Williams BR, Ponesse JS, Schachar RJ, et al. Development of inhibitory control across the life span. Dev Psychol 1999;35(1):205–13.

36. Sweeney GM, Donovan CL, March S, et al. Logging into therapy: adolescent perceptions of online therapies for mental health problems. Internet Interv 2016. https://doi.org/10.1016/j.invent.2016.12.001.

Avoidant/Restrictive Food Intake Disorder

Rachel Bryant-Waugh, BSc, MSc, DPhil

KEYWORDS

- ARFID • Avoidant/restrictive food intake disorder • Feeding disorders
- Restrictive eating disorders • Children • Adolescents

KEY POINTS

- Prevalence and incidence rates of avoidant/restrictive food intake disorder (ARFID) in the general population remain largely unknown. Reliable screening instruments are needed to progress with this information.
- Despite ongoing variability in the interpretation of diagnostic criteria in clinical practice, good progress has been made regarding recognition and assessment of ARFID.
- Different approaches to treatment are currently being explored; emerging evidence suggests that a range of treatment modalities targeting specific presenting features may be required.
- Reported outcomes for ARFID vary, consistent with the heterogeneity of the disorder. At present, there is insufficient evidence to determine the likely course and prognosis.
- Future directions for research could be usefully informed by closer collaboration with other fields, including feeding disorders, emotion processing and regulation, neurodevelopment, and appetite.

INTRODUCTION

Since its 2013 introduction as a formal diagnostic category in the American Psychiatric Association's *Diagnostic and Statistical Manual of Mental Disorders* (DSM), 5th edition,[1] avoidant/restrictive food intake disorder (ARFID) has been widely accepted as a recognized condition. Clinical and research interest has grown, with an increasing number of publications documenting a range of aspects of its presentation. This level of attention is greater than that afforded to ARFID's predecessor in DSM-IV: the diagnostic category feeding disorder of infancy or early childhood.[2] This attracted only limited research interest and was generally regarded as having

The author has no disclosures to declare of any relationship with a commercial company that has a direct financial interest in subject matter or materials discussed in this article or with a company making a competing product.

Population, Policy and Practice Programme, UCL Great Ormond Street Institute of Child Health, 30 Guilford Street, London, WC1N 1EH, UK

E-mail address: r.bryant-waugh@ucl.ac.uk

Child Adolesc Psychiatric Clin N Am 28 (2019) 557–565
https://doi.org/10.1016/j.chc.2019.05.004
1056-4993/19/© 2019 Elsevier Inc. All rights reserved.

limited clinical utility.[3] ARFID arose out of evidence supporting this view, with the proposed and eventually accepted diagnostic criteria based on data highlighting the existence of clinically significant avoidant or restrictive food intake behaviors in children, adolescents, and adults. Several of these presentations have been well described, with evidence suggesting they were distinguishable from the eating disorders anorexia nervosa (AN) and bulimia nervosa, as well as other mental or behavioral disorders.[4] Further support to introduce ARFID as a diagnostic category came from the workup to the 11th revision of the World Health Organization's *International Statistical Classification of Diseases and Related Health Problems* (ICD).[5,6] As a result, ARFID is now included in both the main diagnostic classification schemes of DSM-5 and ICD-11.

In the time since ARFID's introduction, several published articles have reflected on this process, summarized what is known, and highlighted the many gaps in knowledge. Overall, research efforts to date have broadly substantiated the recognition of ARFID as a distinct diagnosis.[7] Current consensus suggests that ARFID involves a heterogeneous cause, is often complex in nature, and can require multidisciplinary input.[8,9] Given the length of time needed to accumulate a robust body of research that can help to determine cause, inform reliable evaluation approaches, tailor treatments, and understand course, several investigators have provided practical overviews to assist clinicians with recognition and general guidance.[10] In relation to youth, clinicians most likely to encounter patients with ARFID are those working in pediatric medical settings, as well as those specializing in mental health.

ARFID seems to have become a focus of attention for those working in the eating disorder field more than for those in the pediatric feeding disorder field,[11] with a few notable exceptions.[12] This is perhaps unsurprising because ARFID now covers several presentations previously included in the large number of patients seen in eating disorder programs with a DSM-IV diagnosis of eating disorder not otherwise specified. This was a sizable, heterogeneous, residual category long recognized as including most of those seeking help for an eating disorder.[13] Many working in pediatric feeding disorders tended not to use the DSM-IV category of feeding disorder of infancy or early childhood; pediatric feeding disorders are not all mental disorders and a psychiatric diagnosis is not relevant or appropriate in many cases. This divergence between the 2 fields, which both concern eating behavior, seems unhelpful because it seems likely that each could learn from the other, to the benefit of patient care. Greater recognition of opportunities and benefits afforded by closer collaboration between the 2 fields is now beginning to emerge.[14]

EPIDEMIOLOGY

Knowledge about the incidence and prevalence of any disorder is fundamental to furthering understanding and planning health care provision. Epidemiologic research explores the distribution of disorders and enables tracking of changes in the numbers affected, as well as the identification of high-risk groups. Knowing if there are particular populations that are more likely to develop ARFID, or key demographic features associated with its incidence, could provide valuable insight into potential determinants. Reliable knowledge about the occurrence of ARFID will depend, as with other disorders, on the representativeness of the populations studied and the methods and measures used to determine its presence. At present, only limited data are available.[15]

Work on identifying ARFID-like presentations in nonclinical cohorts includes a study of Swiss children aged 8 to 13 years. The project set out to determine the distribution of restrictive eating disturbances characteristic of ARFID in this age group, and also to evaluate a newly developed screening instrument: the Eating Disturbances in Youth-Questionnaire (EDY-Q).[16] This is a 12-item self-report measure, based on DSM-5 diagnostic criteria for ARFID.[1] Of 1444 participants screened, 46 (3.2%) self-identified features of ARFID. The investigators note that underweight children reported features of ARFID more often than normal and overweight children. It is not possible to be certain whether these individuals would have met formal diagnostic criteria for ARFID. Nevertheless, the EDY-Q is reported as performing satisfactorily in terms of psychometric properties and thus represents a potentially useful tool to continue to evaluate.[17] A further population-based survey, conducted in Australia, reported on the prevalence and burden of ARFID (as well as other eating disorders) in adolescents older than the age of 15 years and adults. Participants were interviewed in 2014 (n = 2732) and 2015 (n = 3005) to obtain demographic information, as well as responses relating to a range of eating disorder diagnoses, including diagnostic criteria for ARFID. In 2014, a 3-month prevalence of ARFID of 0.3% (95% CI 0.1–0.5) was reported. In 2015, this was 0.3% (95% CI 0.2–0.6). These are marginally lower than the figures obtained for AN. Mental health–related quality of life was found to be particularly poor in the ARFID group, who additionally had lower role performance (ie, the ability to fulfill responsibilities at home, school, or work) than those without an eating disorder.[18] These findings are of interest but they do not provide a complete picture. Children and younger adolescents were not included and this is the age group in whom ARFID presentations have been most frequently and most consistently described. This study does, however, highlight the potential for significant negative impact of ARFID, also identified by other investigators.

A surveillance study collaboration across Australia, Canada, and the United Kingdom reports further useful data. In each country, pediatricians and child psychiatrists were asked to report symptoms of any child younger than 12 years with a newly diagnosed restrictive eating disorder over a defined period (36, 24, and 14 months for the above-mentioned countries, respectively). Descriptive and latent class analyses were performed for each country separately, then compared. Results revealed 2 clusters: 1 resembling AN and the other resembling ARFID. Participants in the latter were more likely to be younger and present with a comorbid psychiatric disorder.[19] A further population-based study of restrictive eating behaviors in 799 7 to 14 year old children in Germany, also using latent class analysis, revealed a 3-cluster solution across all age groups. These included an asymptomatic class, a class with restrictive eating behaviors without shape concern (resembling ARFID), and a class showing restrictive eating behaviors with prominent shape concern (resembling AN).[20] Findings suggesting 2 distinct phenotypes are mirrored by several studies investigating the prevalence of ARFID in adolescent eating disorder programs and conducting comparisons between diagnostic groups. In these settings, ARFID patients have generally been identified as, on average, younger; having higher rates of both psychiatric and medical comorbidities; and more likely to be male than other eating disorder patients.[21–25] Finally, another study set out to identify the prevalence in a pediatric treatment-seeking sample attending gastroenterology clinics in the United States (n = 2231 aged 8–18 years). It was hypothesized that some features of ARFID would be common, yet cases found to meet full criteria were found to be relatively rare at 1.5% of the total screened.[26] Again, the identified cases were predominantly male and the findings support ARFID as a distinct construct.

In conclusion, comprehensive epidemiologic data in fully representative populations remain very limited. Several screening measures have been proposed for ARFID, or are currently in development.[27] Published incidence and prevalence data are scarce and no single screening measure has yet emerged as superior in relation to capturing the full range of ARFID presentations in either clinical or nonclinical populations.

CLINICAL ASSESSMENT AND DIAGNOSIS

ARFID is now widely recognized as a multifaceted disorder that may arise from a range of potential contributing factors and carry varying levels of risk. Multidisciplinary assessment has been recommended,[14] in part because of the need to rule out any medical or psychiatric conditions that may directly account for the eating disturbance but also because treatment may require the input of clinicians from a range of different disciplines. Weight may be low, normal, or high, and there may be significant nutritional compromise, which can be missed if the patient is normal weight.[28] The potential for cultural challenges to assessment and diagnosis has also been raised; however, to date, the role of culture in the development and expression of ARFID has not yet been adequately studied.[29]

DSM-5 diagnostic criteria for ARFID currently include 3 examples of contributing factors that may underlie the eating disturbance: low interest in food or eating, avoidance based on the sensory characteristics of food, and concern about possible aversive consequences of eating.[1] Although some investigators have interpreted this to mean there are 3 ARFID subtypes, this has not yet been established. Further work in this area would be helpful because it seems likely that optimal treatment may vary depending on specific features of presentation.[30,31]

Standardized assessment measures can aid consistency in describing presenting features, as well as improving reliability, of diagnosis. It has been observed that many psychometric measures in routine use in eating disorder settings are not sufficiently specific to allow a diagnosis of ARFID to be made and may not be sensitive as assessment tools.[25] To address this, several groups have been developing new measures to include those for use with youth in clinical settings. These include the Eating Disorder Assessment for DSM-5 (EDA-5),[32] the Eating Disorder Examination–ARFID (EDE-ARFID) module,[33] and the Pica, ARFID, and Rumination Disorder Interview (PARDI).[34] As with screening instruments, the performance of these measures on a wider scale remains to be established but, at this stage, all seem promising. The EDA-5 is a diagnostic instrument, whereas the EDE-ARFID module and the PARDI provide more detailed clinical information, as well as diagnostic algorithms. Additionally, the PARDI is available in multiinformant formats.[34]

TREATMENT

Several published clinical descriptions, review papers, and research reports contribute to knowledge about current medical and psychological treatment approaches for ARFID. To date, available evidence for specific modalities should, at best, be regarded as preliminary, with a clear indication that multimodal, multidisciplinary input may be required. Further research is undoubtedly needed to determine optimal treatment modalities for different presentations of ARFID.[35–37] A survey carried out with adolescent medicine specialists and other physicians in the United States demonstrated significant variability in current practice when caring for hospitalized patients with ARFID.[38] Some such patients are treated alongside those with AN, using similar protocols, although the efficacy of the latter has not been established formally with ARFID patients. It would seem likely that AN treatment protocols have the potential to assist with weight gain. However, given that not all ARFID patients present with low weight and the significant differences in psychopathology between the 2 disorders, these should not be considered sufficient or accepted practice. More information about longer term outcomes is needed to determine whether existing approaches for other eating disorders are helpful, inconclusive, or indeed harmful for those with ARFID.

Single case studies, case series, and nonrandomized clinical trials of psychological approaches have so far predominantly investigated or reported on behavioral, cognitive behavioral, and family-based interventions for children and adolescents with ARFID.[37,39–41] There are as yet no published results from any randomized controlled treatment trial for any intervention. However, results have been published for a small pilot study investigating the feasibility and preliminary efficacy of an intensive, manual-based behavioral feeding intervention for young children with ARFID.[12] The investigators concluded that the results are promising and warrant a large-scale randomized trial to test the safety and efficacy of this approach.[12] An important additional study, not yet published, is a randomized controlled cross-over trial testing the feasibility and acceptability of a novel intervention: family-based treatment of ARFID in children with ARFID aged 5 to 12 years.[42,43]

Several different medications have also been reported as possible adjunctive treatment approaches for ARFID, with positive outcomes noted in some patients taking olanzapine, fluoxetine, and/or cyproheptadine.[41] It is not possible to determine specific medication effects in most reports, given its administration alongside other treatment components. Cyproheptadine has previously been identified as safe and effective for use in young children with eating difficulties related to low appetite, again, as an adjunct to specialized multidisciplinary intervention.[44] One study, comparing ARFID subjects on low doses of olanzapine to those not taking medication in a child and adolescent eating disorders program, concluded that, used in this way, olanzapine may improve eating, weight gain, and the reduction of anxious, depressive, and cognitive symptoms, and thus warrants further study.[45] A further recent, double-blind, placebo-controlled trial of 15 children aged 20 to 58 months with a diagnosis of ARFID compared behavioral intervention with behavioral intervention plus D-cycloserine (DCS). DCS has previously been shown to facilitate exposure interventions in anxiety disorders.[46] Due to observed improvements to eating behavior in the DCS group, the investigators conclude that the positive results noted warrant a larger scale study of DCS for treatment of pediatric feeding problems, to include ARFID.[46] Due to its efficacy in adult anxiety and depression, mirtazapine has also been put forward as a potentially useful drug to evaluate in the treatment of ARFID. However, the investigators note that there is only limited research on the use of mirtazapine in children and adolescents generally, and that it is off-label for pediatric populations.[47] Future randomized, placebo-controlled studies in ARFID may be warranted but, at present, there is insufficient evidence to support any medication as a first-line treatment intervention.

PROGNOSIS AND OUTCOME

As with most aspects of ARFID there has been limited research on prognosis, course, and outcome so that any statements or predictions in this respect must be tentative. A few findings are beginning to emerge, including the observation by some investigators that a small number of ARFID patients may go on to be classified AN as treatment progresses.[21] It is difficult to be certain whether this represents a possible trajectory in the course of the disorder or whether these subjects may have been misclassified initially. Other investigators report on short-term treatment outcomes following in-patient admission alongside other subjects with eating disorders.[48] One study identified greater reliance on enteral feeding and longer lengths of stay in ARFID patients compared with AN patients.[49] Again, the interpretation of such findings is difficult; if the treatment is not optimally targeting specific features of ARFID, it may be less likely to be effective. One study including ARFID subjects receiving partial hospitalization treatment in the context of low weight found that weight gain was maintained at 12-month follow-up but ongoing outpatient treatment was required in most after discharge.[50] Finally, a retrospective study including 700 subjects with restrictive eating disorders from 14 different adolescent medicine eating disorder programs in the United States identified 12.4% (N = 87) with ARFID. At 1-year follow-up, these subjects showed no difference from other diagnostic groups in terms of positive change in mean percentage median body mass index, with the main predictor of weight change being weight at admission.[51] These findings suggest that, overall, eating disorder programs are skilled at supporting young people with restrictive eating disorders to gain weight, but they do not provide much detail about the longer term prognosis of ARFID in particular. This is particularly important because low weight is not necessarily a defining feature of ARFID. One of the few studies with longer term outcome data of potential interest, is a longitudinal study following 113 children with ARFID-like presentations (characterized by low interest in eating) from the age of 2 through to 11 years. The investigators report evidence of enduring risk of malnutrition and increasing psychopathological symptoms.[52]

FUTURE DIRECTIONS

ARFID is now established as a distinct disorder based on consistent evidence supporting differences in clinical presentation with the other eating disorders. This has been further strengthened by population-based studies, which also suggest that there are differences between restrictive eating behaviors associated with weight or shape concern and those occurring in the absence of such concerns. Research into ARFID is now picking up, with much needed attention being paid to some of the many gaps in knowledge. Treatment research is essential; however, to ensure this is appropriately directed, further exploration and testing of etiologic and maintaining models is required. At present, recommendations regarding treatment are primarily based on existing treatment protocols for eating disorders, with or without some modification. Clinical experience, also from the feeding disorders field, and identification of putative maintaining factors on an individual basis, with delivery of appropriate evidence-based treatment approaches are also used. More sophisticated understanding of the psychopathology of the full range of ARFID presentations is required to ensure optimally targeted psychological interventions.

In seeking to progress in the field of ARFID in children and adolescents, it will be important to remain alert, not only to emerging knowledge and developments in the wider eating disorders field but also in the arenas of pediatric feeding disorders, anxiety and related emotion processing and regulation, neurodevelopment, and psychobiological approaches to appetite and eating behavior. Postulated explanatory models are beginning to emerge, such as a 3-dimensional model hypothesizing neurobiological abnormalities in sensory perception, homeostatic appetite, and negative valence systems.[53] At present, however, such models have not been adequately tested and their treatment implications remain unknown.

Several significant challenges remain, not least in terms of precise characterization of the disorder for research purposes and ascertaining the scale of the problem in population terms. Given the multiple routes leading to food avoidance or restriction, and the presence of dimensional differences between caseness and normal variation in many aspects of eating behavior, there is a way to go. On the plus side, knowledge about ARFID is increasing all the time and the interested reader is well-advised to keep track of the literature to remain fully informed.

REFERENCES

1. American Psychiatric Association. Diagnostic and statistical manual of mental disorders. 5th edition. Arlington (VA): American Psychiatric Publishing; 2013.
2. American Psychiatric Association. Diagnostic and statistical manual of mental disorders. 4th edition, text rev. Arlington (VA): American Psychiatric Publishing; 2013.
3. Kenney L, Walsh BT. Avoidant/restrictive food intake disorder (ARFID). Eating Disorders Review 2013;24:1–4.
4. Bryant-Waugh R, Markham L, Kreipe RE, et al. Feeding and eating disorders in childhood. Int J Eat Disord 2010;43:98–111.
5. Uher R, Rutter M. Classification of feeding and eating disorders: review of evidence and proposals for ICD-11. World Psychiatry 2012;11:80–92.
6. Available at: https://icd.who.int/browse11/l-m/en#/http://id.who.int/icd/entity/1242188600. Accessed November 27, 2018.
7. Norris ML, Katzman DK. Change is never easy, but it is possible: reflections on avoidant/restrictive food intake disorder two years after its introduction in the DSM-5. J Adolesc Health 2015;57:8–9.
8. Zimmerman J, Fisher M. Avoidant/restrictive food intake disorder (ARFID). Curr Probl Pediatr Adolesc Health Care 2017;47:95–103.
9. Mairs R, Nicholls D. Assessment and treatment of eating disorders in children and adolescents. Arch Dis Child 2016;101:1168–75.
10. Mammel KA, Ornstein RA. Avoidant/restrictive food intake disorder: a new eating disorder diagnosis in the Diagnostic and Statistical Manual 5. Curr Opin Pediatr 2017;29:407–13.
11. Kennedy GA, Wick MR, Keel PK. Eating disorders in children: is avoidant-restrictive food intake disorder a feeding disorder or an eating disorder and what are the implications for treatment? F1000Res 2018;7:88.
12. Sharp WG, Stubbs KH, Adams H, et al. Intensive, manual-based intervention for pediatric feeding disorders: results from a randomized pilot trial. J Pediatr Gastroenterol Nutr 2016;62:658–63.
13. Fairburn C, Bohn K. Eating disorder NOS (EDNOS): an example of the troublesome "not otherwise specified" (NOS) category in DSM-IV. Behav Res Ther 2005;43:691–701.
14. Eddy KT, Harshman SG, Becker KR, et al. Radcliffe ARFID Workgroup: Commentary on diagnosis, multi-disciplinary assessment and treatment, and directions for the field. Int J Eat Disord 2019;52:361–6.
15. Lindvall Dahlgren C, Wisting L, Rø Ø. Feeding and eating disorders in the DSM-5 era: a systematic review of prevalence rates in non-clinical male and female samples. J Eat Disord 2017;5:56.
16. Kurz S, van Dyck Z, Dremmel D, et al. Early-onset restrictive eating disturbances in primary school boys and girls. Eur Child Adolesc Psychiatry 2015;24:779–85.
17. Kurz S, van Dyck Z, Dremmel D, et al. Variants of early-onset restrictive eating disturbances in middle childhood. Int J Eat Disord 2016;49:102–6.
18. Hay P, Mitchison D, Collado AEL. Burden and health-related quality of life of eating disorders, including Avoidant/Restrictive Food Intake Disorder (ARFID), in the Australian population. J Eat Disord 2017;5:21.

19. Pinhas L, Nicholls D, Crosby RD, et al. Classification of childhood onset eating disorders: a latent class analysis. Int J Eat Disord 2017;50:657–64.
20. Schmidt R, Vogel M, Hiemisch A, et al. Pathological and non-pathological variants of restrictive eating behaviors in middle childhood: a latent class analysis. Appetite 2018;127:257–65.
21. Norris ML, Robinson A, Obeid N. Exploring avoidant/restrictive food intake disorder in eating disordered patients: a descriptive study. Int J Eat Disord 2014;47: 495–9.
22. Norris ML, Spettigue WJ, Katzman DK. Update on eating disorders: current perspectives on avoidant/restrictive food intake disorder in children and youth. Neuropsychiatr Dis Treat 2016;12:213–8.
23. Fisher MM, Rosen DS, Ornstein RM, et al. Characteristics of avoidant/restrictive food intake disorder in children and adolescents: a "new disorder" in DSM-5. J Adolesc Health 2014;55:49–52.
24. Nicely TA, Lane-Loney S, Masciulli E, et al. Prevalence and characteristics of avoidant/restrictive food intake disorder in a cohort of young patients in day treatment for eating disorders. J Eat Disord 2014;2:21.
25. Cooney M, Lieberman M, Guimond, et al. Clinical and psychological features of children and adolescents diagnosed with avoidant/restrictive food intake disorder in a pediatric tertiary care eating disorder program: a descriptive study. J Eat Disord 2018;6:7.
26. Eddy KT, Thomas JJ, Hastings E, et al. Prevalence of DSM-5 avoidant/restrictive food intake disorder in a pediatric gastroenterology healthcare network. Int J Eat Disord 2015;48:464–70.
27. Zickgraf HF, Ellis M. Initial validation of the Nine Item Avoidant/Restrictive Food Intake disorder screen (NIAS): a measure of three restrictive eating patterns. Appetite 2018;123:32–42.
28. Chandran JJ, Anderson G, Kennedy A, et al. Subacute combined degeneration of the spinal cord in an adolescent male with avoidant/restrictive food intake disorder: a clinical case report. Int J Eat Disord 2015;48:1176–9.
29. Shermbrucker J, Kimber M, JohnsonN, et al. Avoidant/restrictive food intake disorder in an 11-year old south american boy: medical and cultural challenges. J Can Acad Child Adolesc Psychiatry 2017;26:110–3.
30. Norris ML, Spettigue W, Hammond NG, et al. Building evidence for the use of descriptive subtypes in youth with avoidant restrictive food intake disorder. Int J Eat Disord 2018;51:170–3.
31. Ornstein RM, Essayli H, Nicely TA, et al. Treatment of avoidant/restrictive food intake disorder in a cohort of young patients in a partial hospitalization program for eating disorders. Int J Eat Disord 2017;50:1067–74.
32. Sysko R, Glasofer DR, Hildebrandt T, et al. The eating disorder assessment for DSM-5 (EDA-5): development and validation of a structured interview for feeding and eating disorders. Int J Eat Disord 2015;48:452–63.
33. Schmidt R, Kirsten T, Hiemisch A, et al. Interview-based assessment of avoidant/ restrictive food intake disorder (ARFID): a pilot study evaluating an ARFID module for the eating disorder examination. Int J Eat Disord 2019;52:388–97.
34. Bryant-Waugh R, Micali N, Cooke L, et al. Development of the Pica, ARFID, and Rumination Disorder Interview, a multi-informant, semi-structured interview of feeding disorders across the lifespan: a pilot study for ages 10-22. Int J Eat Disord 2019;52:378–87.
35. Herpertz-Dahlmann B. Treatment of eating disorders in child and adolescent psychiatry. Curr Opin Psychiatry 2017;30:438–45.

36. Lock J. An update on evidence-based psychosocial treatments for eating disorders in children and adolescents. J Clin Child Adolesc Psychol 2015;44:707–21.
37. Thomas JJ, Wons OB, Eddy KT, et al. Cognitive-behavioral treatment of avoidant/restrictive food intake disorder. Curr Opin Psychiatry 2018;31:425–30.
38. Guss CE, Richmond TK, Forman S. A survey of physician practices on the inpatient medical stabilization of patients with avoidant/restrictive food intake disorder. J Eat Disord 2018;6:22.
39. Pitt PD, Middleman AB. A focus on behavior management of avoidant/restrictive food intake disorder (ARFID): a case series. Clin Pediatr (Phila) 2018;57:478–80.
40. Bryant-Waugh R. Avoidant restrictive food intake disorder: an illustrative case example. Int J Eat Disord 2013;46:420–3.
41. Spettigue W, Norris ML, Santos A, et al. Treatment of children and adolescents with avoidant/restrictive food intake disorder: a case series examining the feasibility of family therapy and adjunctive treatments. J Eat Disord 2018;6:20.
42. Lock J. Treating ARFID using family-based treatment: a randomized controlled crossover trial. Available at: https://www.nationaleatingdisorders.org/ways-to-give/feeding-hope-fund-clinical-research/recipients/. Accessed August 15, 2018.
43. Rienecke RD. Family based treatment of eating disorders in adolescents: current insights. Adolesc Health Med Ther 2017;8:69–79.
44. Sant'Anna AM, Hammes PS, Porporino M, et al. Use of cyproheptadine in young children with feeding difficulties and poor growth in a pediatric feeding program. J Pediatr Gastroenterol Nutr 2014;59:674–8.
45. Brewerton TD, D'Agostino M. Adjunctive use of olanzapine in the treatment of avoidant/restrictive food intake disorder in children and adolescents in an eating disorders program. J Child Adolesc Psychopharmacol 2017;27:920–2.
46. Sharp WG, Allen AG, Stubbs KH, et al. Successful pharmacotherapy for the treatment of severe feeding aversion with mechanistic insights from cross-species neuronal remodelling. Transl Psychiatry 2017;7:1157.
47. Gray E, Chen T, Menzel J, et al. Mirtazapine and weight gain in avoidant and restrictive food intake disorder. J Am Acad Child Adolesc Psychiatry 2018;57:288–9.
48. Peebles R, Lesser A, Park CC, et al. Outcomes of an inpatient medical nutritional rehabilitation protocol in children and adolescents with eating disorders. J Eat Disord 2017;5:7.
49. Strandjord SE, Sieke EH, Richmond M, et al. Avoidant/restrictive food intake disorder: illness and hospital course in patients hospitalized for nutritional insufficiency. J Adolesc Health 2015;57:673–8.
50. Bryson AE, Scipioni AM, Essayli JH, et al. Outcomes of low-weight patients with avoidant/restrictive food intake disorder and anorexia nervosa at long-term follow-up after treatment in a partial hospitalization program for eating disorders. Int J Eat Disord 2018;51:470–4.
51. Forman SF, McKenzie N, Hehn R, et al. Predictors of outcome at 1 year in adolescents with DSM-5 restrictive eating disorders: report of the national eating disorders quality improvement collaborative. J Adolesc Health 2014;55:750–6.
52. Lucarelli L, Sechi C, Cimino S, et al. Avoidant/restrictive food intake disorder: a longitudinal study of malnutrition and psychopathological risk factors from 2 to 11 Years of age. Front Psychol 2018;9:1608.
53. Thomas JJ, Lawson EA, Micali N, et al. Avoidant/restrictive food intake disorder: a three-dimensional model of neurobiology with implications for etiology and treatment. Curr Psychiatry Rep 2017;19:54.

Eating Disorders in Transitional Age Youth

Jennifer Derenne, MD

KEYWORDS

- Eating disorders • Anorexia nervosa • Bulimia nervosa • Transitional age youth
- College student mental health

KEY POINTS

- Earlier identification and better treatment have allowed more students to matriculate at institutions of higher learning, but students' needs have stretched available university resources.
- Given the prevalence of disordered eating in the college population, most universities have clinicians with expertise in this area on staff. However, there is wide variability in the services available on campus, and this must be taken into account when students are making decisions on where they would like to attend school.
- Some students find it necessary to take a gap year before matriculation to cement medical and psychological stability. Others may find it helpful to start in a community college setting, or to start out living at home with a reduced course load in order to optimize chances for success. Still others may decide on different pathways such as the military, a volunteer experience, or joining the workforce directly after high school.
- Parents have more influence than they may realize over an adult child's treatment decisions. Although it is true that the individual has the right to refuse treatment once he or she reaches the age of majority, parents also have the right to make ongoing financial support contingent on the individual's health and participation in appropriate medical and psychiatric treatment.
- Evidence-based treatments, such as family-based treatment (FBT), can be modified for use in transitional age youth to take developmental issues into account while also providing the accountability and support likely necessary to promote full and lasting recovery from an eating disorder.

Eating disorder treatment, although challenging under the best circumstances, becomes even more difficult in the setting of the transition to adulthood. Once individuals turn 18, outpatient clinicians and programs providing higher levels of care require that they enroll in treatment voluntarily. Parents struggle to know how much they can push

Disclosure: The author has nothing to disclose.
Division of Child and Adolescent Psychiatry, Stanford University School of Medicine, 401 Quarry Road, Stanford, CA 94304, USA
E-mail address: jderenne@stanford.edu

Child Adolesc Psychiatric Clin N Am 28 (2019) 567–572
https://doi.org/10.1016/j.chc.2019.05.010
childpsych.theclinics.com

or insist on given their child's new found legal rights. Patients, too, can be challenged to anticipate their treatment needs, particularly when starting a job or making the transition to college. Although growing up and becoming more independent is exciting for many, it can also present significant challenges, with individuals often wanting to "start fresh," without the need for ongoing treatment relationships. Many emerging adults want desperately to "stay in step" with peers who are making similar transitions, but may fail to appreciate the complexities of balancing treatment with living independently, negotiating adult relationships, and taking on more autonomy with respect to academic endeavors.

Over the past few years, colleges and universities have seen an increase in students requesting mental health support.[1] The upside is that this seems to indicate that earlier identification of mental health concerns and better treatment interventions have allowed more young people the opportunity to matriculate at institutes of higher learning. It may also suggest that stigma plays less of a role in the decision to seek treatment than it has in the past. It also means, however, that colleges and universities, who have not always been able to add additional mental health staff, have struggled to meet the needs of students with more specialized mental health treatment needs. According to the American College Health Association's biannual study in spring of 2018, 28.1% of students self-identify as having anxiety and 19.8% report depression requiring ongoing treatment. Over the preceding year, 1.6% report a diagnosis of anorexia nervosa, and 1.2% report a diagnosis of bulimia nervosa. Eighteen percent of students feel that mental health concerns have affected their ability to study or to manage work expectations. A total of 7.8% report feeling so distressed that they have considered suicide.[2]

The college environment can promote disordered eating in many important ways. Some young people have never had to plan or prepare meals for themselves, and may get overwhelmed with the options available in the campus cafeteria. Some buffet style offerings promote binge eating, whereas others are only open at certain hours that may not coincide with the student's course schedule. Some students take a keen interest in nutrition and may find it difficult to consume food that they have not prepared themselves. Many arrive at school with a desire to be attractive to peers and potential romantic partners, and a worry about gaining the "freshmen fifteen." Some are used to playing on school or club sports teams and having a regular exercise schedule that disappears when starting classes. Others use exercise to manage stress and anxiety, and may find it difficult to eat regularly when stressed or overwhelmed.[3]

Many young people with a history of disordered eating are college bound. Patients living with anorexia nervosa, for example, tend to cite perfectionism, the desire for achievement, and holding oneself to high standards as characteristics that allow them to be successful but also can make it challenging to let go of the cognitive rigidity that underlies many eating disorders. For this reason, and for the simple fact that eating disorders commonly present in this age group, clinicians practicing at College Counseling and Student Health Centers tend to see eating disorders, and many university health centers have eating disorder specialists on staff. Some even convene multidisciplinary treatment teams to streamline care and improve communication among therapists, psychiatrists, physicians, and dietitians.[4] However, it is important to recognize that university mental health services are not standardized. In fact, they are quite variable, and the availability of specialty resources such as those necessary for treating eating disorders may be limited by geographic location. For example, a college or university in a major city is much more likely to have specialty eating disorder treatment resources in close proximity compared with an institution located in a more rural area. Access to services such as partial hospital programs or intensive outpatient programs can be important for students who struggle without external structure and support. It is also important to note that some college counseling centers have limits on the number of sessions available (often 10 or less) for on-campus counseling and may limit these visits to those necessary to process homesickness, roommate challenges, breakups, or difficulties managing academics and learning study skills. Some dictate that those patients with chronic conditions requiring specialty care must be referred and managed off campus. Clearly, these are limitations that are essential for families and referring clinicians to explore before making a decision about college choice.

In addition, it is important for families to consider several other factors when making decisions about where to go to college. For example, how far away from home is reasonable? Are there extended family members or friends nearby who could be called on to help in the event of a health emergency? What happens if the student begins to struggle despite having a solid treatment plan in place? Does the student have any other co-morbid mental health conditions that may affect their transition, such as separation anxiety or depression? Do they have the experience to know whether they might be prone to homesickness? Have they had the practice of managing sleep and wake cycles, getting themselves up in the morning on time for class, and managing schedules and deadlines without a lot of external support from parents, coaches, tutors, and teachers? Although it may sound trivial, it is actually important for students to know how to do laundry, make and keep appointments, fill prescriptions, and manage a budget, and resist the temptation to sleep late, skip class, play video games, and stay up late socializing with friends. Substance use and abuse are rampant in the college population, and patients with eating disorders may be particularly at risk for misusing stimulant medications to manage weight and appetite concerns, while also optimizing their productivity during study time. In addition, the binge drinking that is so common on college campuses can lead to excess caloric consumption due to the intake of alcohol itself, combined with decreased inhibition that may lead to over-eating and compensatory strategies to avoid weight gain.

Students with eating concerns may present in many ways. Some will self-refer with medical or psychological concerns, whereas others will seek medical attention for malaise, poor energy, vague gastrointestinal complaints, amenorrhea, or sexual concerns. At times, a student will come to the attention of the residence life office after another student expresses concern about his or her unhealthy eating and exercise habits. Faculty members may express concern about a student's significant weight loss. Environmental services may raise a red flag about suspected purging after repeated calls to service clogged toilets and drains. Staff at the recreation center may become concerned about students spending hours at the gym each day, or cafeteria workers may notice students with unusual eating patterns.

Even on campuses with access to the most appropriate treatment resources, there are many barriers to treatment. Stigma and shame are high on the list, as is denial by students who normalize or minimize their behavior. Students are notoriously busy and may find it challenging to make time in their schedules for necessary appointments, particularly around high-stress times such as midterms and finals (which are also the times when support for disordered eating is likely to be most needed). Cost is another real issue. College student health insurance programs may limit coverage for specialized eating disorder treatment. Some campuses allow students to sign waivers allowing them to opt out of the student health insurance coverage; many remain covered on their parents' policy until age 26 years, but others choose to forego coverage altogether, with the rationale that they are young and otherwise healthy.

Community specialty providers may not work with insurance, which adds significant cost to a student budget. Finally, some students worry that seeking treatment on campus will affect their academic record and may affect their ability to apply to graduate or professional school in the future. It is important for students and families to understand that health and academic records are kept separate, and that seeking treatment for a health condition will not appear on the academic transcript. This is especially important for families trying to determine whether to inform the school about eating disorder treatment. Although the decision is ultimately one that needs to be made by the student and parents, it may be of help for them to know that the administration is invested in providing support so that the student can remain enrolled and graduate on schedule.

Getting young adults to acknowledge the need for assessment and treatment can be challenging, and fraught with ethical concerns. Adults have the right to make decisions about their health and treatment, and do have the right to privacy while at college, which is outlined in the Family Educational Rights and Privacy Act, and protects educational records. At the same time, there is a societal expectation that universities abide by the principle of *in loco parentis* and that they will intervene if there is significant concern about health or safety. The Americans with Disabilities Act stipulates that universities cannot discriminate against a student based on a medical or psychiatric diagnosis. However, they do have the right (and the obligation to other members of the university community) to make sure that behaviors do not disrupt the campus or put health or safety at risk. For this reason, many universities maintain a Student of Concern team that meets regularly to discuss how to manage problematic student behavior. These teams are generally made up of representatives from the College Counseling and Student Health Centers, the Dean of Students, the head of Security, Residence Life, and the general counsel. Colleges may require that a student undergo a mandated assessment and treatment if there is significant concern about health, and they may choose to make an exception to confidentiality and inform a student's family about the situation if needed. Failure to comply with recommendations could result in the university proceeding with an involuntary medical leave. Although some students believe that these actions are punitive, most universities take these decisions seriously, and proceed thoughtfully. Generally, the student is closely followed by the team until the treatment providers indicate that the student's condition has stabilized, and then the frequency of contact tapers.[1]

Not all emerging adults choose to attend college. Some may decide to volunteer, travel, join the military, or to enter the workforce directly. In these individuals, refusal to seek care is even more challenging to manage given that there is not an institution, such as a university, to make continued enrollment contingent on participating in treatment and following recommendations. In these situations, parents are often in the difficult position of needing to enforce limits to keep their child healthy. Although it is true that an 18-year-old has a legal right to choose to participate in treatment, parents have more influence than they may think. They are likely still providing substantial financial and emotional support, which can be used as leverage to encourage the young adult to participate in the necessary treatment. For example, parents do not need to continue to fund cell phone service, car insurance, and college tuition. They are allowed to stipulate that the young adult must be actively working in treatment to attain health as a condition of continuing to live in their home. It can feel hard to enforce these limits, as parents (and their adult children) often feel that they are punishing their child for being ill. However, when framed as giving the young person the motivation to take advantage of life-saving treatment, most parents feel more comfortable enforcing limits. In particularly severe cases, parents have found it necessary to petition the court to attain guardianship to make medical decisions for their adult child.

It is important to note that family-based treatment (FBT), which is the treatment approach with the most evidence to support its use in adolescent anorexia nervosa, has been modified for use in transitional age youth and has evidence to support its use in this population as well. Chen and colleagues[5] looked at the efficacy and acceptability of FBT in 18- to 26-year-old women with anorexia nervosa or atypical anorexia nervosa. FBT was modified to include the following adaptations:

1. Subjects were able to choose a support adult other than a parent.
2. Therapists allowed the young adult more autonomy than would usually be allowed in deciding what and where to eat, and also allowed them to participate in decisions about how best to return to normal activities. However, if they were not able to continue to restore weight, decisions reverted to the support adult.
3. Therapists addressed developmental issues such as transition from high school to college.
4. Individuals were allowed more individual therapy session time without the support adult in the final phase of FBT.

Although there was a fairly high dropout rate (9/22), those who completed treatment found the intervention to be acceptable, and were able to restore weight, with body mass index increases comparable with those found in traditional FBT for adolescents. Interestingly, 14/22 picked a parent to be their support person, even though they were able to select significant others, siblings, roommates, or friends. Dimitropoulos and colleagues[6] similarly looked at FBT-transition age youth, which included 25 sessions of treatment. Participants were allowed to choose any supportive adult, and they were given more individual time with the therapist before the "family" portion of each session. They were allowed to keep some personal content confidential, but weight and other eating disorder-specific concerns were shared with the supportive adult. In the first phase, the patient and supportive adult worked collaboratively to restore weight, with the patient describing how the supportive adult could be most helpful to them. In the second phase, the participant focused on eating independently in developmentally appropriate situations, and, in the third phase, the patient attended several independent sessions to focus on relapse prevention, later sharing their plan with family in hopes of taking the next step to resuming normal life and working toward long-term goals. In this study, 26 patients ages 16 to 25 restored weight and demonstrated improvements on the Eating Disorder Examination Questionnaire at the end of treatment and 3-month follow-up. All elected to involve family in the treatment sessions, although a few also included partners and friends.

When preparing youth for the transition to adulthood, it is important that the treating clinician make sure that the family is aware of the limitations on treatment in college counseling centers. Many times, families are woefully unprepared and disappointed when they realize that necessary supports and resources are not available. Students are much more likely to be successful with the transition if they have been stable for at least a few months before moving out of their parents' home and have had practice being more independent with meal preparation and managing activity while still having oversight from parents and the treatment team. In the months leading up to transition, a detailed relapse prevention plan should be discussed, with clearly delineated contingencies. It is imperative that all involved are willing to follow the guidelines agreed on. For example, if the treatment guidelines stipulate that the young adult will take a medical leave if he or she drops below a certain weight, this will need to happen, even if the student begs for more time or parents feel badly about stressing their child.

The student should also sign release of information forms so that the home treatment team can provide a complete handoff to the team at the school, as well as allowing parents access to the school treatment team providers. This does not mean that all of the details of treatment need to be shared with parents. However, it is really helpful for parents to know if the student starts skipping appointments or experiences a significant loss of weight or change in vital sign stability.

Eating disorder treatment is complex, even under optimal circumstances. Transition to adulthood adds a particularly challenging dynamic, but can be successful with adequate preparation and discussion to determine the most effective treatment plan and safety net.

REFERENCES

1. Martel A, Derenne J, Leebens PK, editors. Promoting safe and effective transitions to college for youth with mental health conditions. Cham, Switzerland: Springer International; 2018.
2. American College Health Association. American College Health Association-National College Health Assessment II: reference group executive summary spring 2018. Silver Spring (MD): American College Health Association; 2018.
3. Derenne J. Successfully launching adolescents with eating disorders to college: the Child and Adolescent Psychiatrist's Perspective. J Am Acad Child Adolesc Psychiatry 2013;52(6).
4. Colborn D, Robinson A. Eating disorders and body image concerns. In: Roberts LW, editor. Student mental health: a guide for psychiatrists, psychologist, and leaders serving in higher education. Washington, DC.: American Psychiatric Association Press; 2018. p. 231–48.
5. Chen EY, Weissman JA, Zeffiro TA, et al. Family-based therapy for young adults with anorexia nervosa restores weight. Int J Eat Disord 2016;49(7):701–7.
6. Dimitropoulos G, Landers A, Freeman V, et al. Open trial of family-based treatment of anorexia nervosa for transition age youth. J Can Acad Child Adolesc Psychiatry 2018;27(10):50–61.

The Role of Higher Levels of Care for Eating Disorders in Youth

Jennifer Derenne, MD

KEYWORDS

- Level of care • Inpatient medical stabilization • Psychiatric hospitalization
- Residential treatment • Partial hospital programs • Intensive outpatient programs

KEY POINTS

- It is always preferable to keep a child or adolescent at home with his or her family for treatment if possible. Family-based treatment allows youth to remain enrolled in school and motivated to return to normal activities while making the behavioral changes necessary to sustain recovery over the long term.
- Medical stabilization in an inpatient setting may be necessary in patients with vital sign instabilities and/or low weight.
- Locked psychiatric units may be necessary in cases of suicidal ideation or self-harm, or to manage behavioral issues such as uncontrolled purging or exercise that are not accompanied by vital sign or laboratory abnormalities.
- The structure of a residential treatment center or partial hospital program may allow an individual to restore weight and make progress with psychological recovery. However, patients are vulnerable to relapse back into patterns of restrictive eating and overexercise unless appropriate oversight and accountability are in place.

For patients with eating disorders who are medically and psychiatrically stable, outpatient treatment is the standard of care. However, there are some patients who require added structure and support due to uncontrolled bingeing and/or purging, compulsive exercise, or inability to take in adequate nutrition to meet needs despite support from family. Other youth may not have family members who are agreeable to providing the accountability and structure necessary to be successful with family-based treatment (FBT). There are several levels of care available, with escalating levels of structure and support.[1] It is generally wise to start with the least restrictive level of care possible and to increase the amount of support as clinically indicated by symptoms and behaviors. Historically, hospitals were able to admit patients for stays of several months.

Dr J. Derenne has no conflicts of interest to disclose.
Division of Child and Adolescent Psychiatry, Stanford University School of Medicine, 401 Quarry Road, Stanford, CA 94304, USA
E-mail address: jderenne@stanford.edu

However, since the 1990s, insurance companies have cut reimbursement for extended hospital stays (longer than 1 month), resulting in the proliferation of niche behavioral programs to provide structure and support for patients requiring more intensive care.

INPATIENT MEDICAL STABILIZATION

Eating disorders have the highest mortality rate of any mental illness, with significant medical comorbidity related to malnutrition.[2] Inpatient medical stabilization is accomplished by rest and increased nutrition, and can occur on general medical-surgical units with consultation from behavioral health and dietetics. Nursing staff are responsible for providing meal support and encouraging rest, which may be a challenge on units without a lot of experience caring for these patients because staff may be unfamiliar with how best to support eating and redirect surreptitious exercise.

Some dedicated medical units provide more specialized milieu treatment: patients with medical complications of malnutrition are grouped together on units that provide group dining support, therapeutic groups, and daily school instruction, in addition to close medical follow-up and psychiatric support. Milieu programs typically offer a comprehensive approach to diagnosis and treatment, and engage a multidisciplinary team to provide optimal care. (See later discussion of such a program.) Teams tend to include a mix of medical providers, psychiatrists, psychologists, dietitians, social workers, case managers, school teachers, art therapists, child life specialists, family health educators, occupational therapists, and chaplains, in addition to nurses and milieu counselors. Families are considered assets in treatment, and patients are encouraged to have supervised meals and snacks with their parents whenever possible so that they can practice eating together while taking advantage of the oversight and support of the team (**Table 1**).

The medical providers initially focus on assessment and workup of other causes of weight loss to rule out additional medical concerns (eg, malignancy, inflammatory bowel disease, celiac sprue, or diabetes), then shift the focus to stabilizing vital signs (particularly bradycardia and orthostasis), correcting laboratory abnormalities, and

Table 1	
Criteria for medical admission for children and adolescents	
Bradycardia	Heart rate <50 during the day Heart rate <45 at night
Hypotension	Blood pressure <90/45 mm Hg
Hypothermia	Temperature <35.6°C or 96°F
Orthostasis (supine for 5 min to standing for 2 min)	Heart rate increases >20 Systolic blood pressure decrease >20 mm Hg Diastolic blood pressure decrease >10 mm Hg
Weight	<75% median body mass index for age and sex
Electrocardiogram abnormalities	Example: prolonged QTc (>460 ms)
Electrolyte abnormalities	Phosphorus <3.0 mg/dL Potassium <3.5 mEq/L Magnesium <1.8 mg/dL
Acute medical events	Examples: syncope, gastrointestinal bleeding, severe dehydration

Adapted from Golden NH, Katzman DK, Sawyer SM, et al. Update on the medical management of eating disorders in adolescents. J Adolesc Health 2015;56(4):372; with permission.

restoring weight in a safe manner while monitoring for evidence of refeeding syndrome.[3]

Patients are initially placed on strict bedrest, which lasts until vital signs begin to improve. They are then able to move about the unit transported by a wheelchair. When vital signs have largely normalized, patients are allowed to move to standard activity, which means that they are allowed to walk to and from unit activities although they are encouraged to remain resting as much as possible. Patients are weighed in a gown each morning after urinating, and urine-specific gravity is checked to assess for waterloading. Vital signs, including orthostatic heart rates and blood pressures, are checked multiple times per day. Bloodwork can be taken daily, if need be, and patients are connected to cardiac telemetry overnight to monitor for dangerously low heart rates or dysrhythmias.

In consultation with the registered dietitian, patients are served a nutritionally balanced meal plan, estimating caloric needs based on age, gender, activity level, and need for weight gain. Meal plans start at 1400 kcal per day, and are advanced as safe and tolerated by approximately 200 kcal per day until goal intake is achieved. Meals are provided at set times, with clear guidelines about timing. Meals last 45 minutes, whereas snacks are 30 minutes. Patients are observed closely to make sure that they are not hiding or microcutting food. They are redirected if they are demonstrating unusual eating behaviors. If they are unwilling or unable to complete all of the solid food in the time allowed, they are given the opportunity to replace the uneaten calories (in a 1:1 ratio) with a nutrition supplement such as Ensure plus. Nasogastric tubes may be necessary in cases of acute food refusal or medical conditions such as superior mesenteric artery syndrome, which limit the rate of feeding.

The psychiatry and psychology team members provide a comprehensive assessment of mental health concerns, including safety, and make the official eating disorder diagnosis. They must also be careful to assess for other mental health conditions that may affect eating and appetite, such as depression, anxiety, psychosis, or obsessive compulsive disorder. Medications, such as stimulants to treat attention-deficit hyperactivity disorder, are known to decrease appetite and may cause weight loss.[4]

During the hospitalization, mental health providers provide psychoeducation about the diagnosis to patients and families, introduce more adaptive coping strategies and relaxation techniques, encourage patients to identify and challenge unhelpful thinking, and assist with aftercare planning. Often, malnourished patients experience physical discomfort with the renourishment process and use techniques such as aromatherapy, diaphragmatic breathing, progressive muscle relaxation, acupressure, and biofeedback to manage this discomfort, rather than relying on large numbers of medications. Some may discharge directly to outpatient therapy such as FBT or adolescent-focused treatment (AFT), whereas others may need or choose to step down to another level of care such as inpatient psychiatry, residential treatment, partial hospitalization, or intensive outpatient treatment.

The role of psychiatric medications is mainly limited to comorbid mood or anxiety disorders that predate the development of the disordered eating.[5] Fluoxetine[6] and lisdexamfetamine[7] do have US Food and Drug Administration indications for adults with bulimia nervosa and binge eating disorder, respectively. In cases in which anxiety or neurovegetative symptoms arose solely in the setting of weight loss and overexercise, it may be prudent to reassess mood and anxiety as renourishment proceeds. The signs and symptoms of malnutrition often mimic those of depression and anxiety. Premeal benzodiazepines are mostly ineffective and may introduce the risk of substance dependence in vulnerable individuals.

Inpatient medical stabilization programs are limited by the rate of medical recovery, which is often faster than that of psychological recovery. Once the patient is no longer considered medically unstable, they must be discharged from the program, even if they are still significantly struggling with intake or urges to purge or exercise. For this reason, it is important to work on aftercare planning from the very start of treatment.

INPATIENT PSYCHIATRIC HOSPITALIZATION

There are 2 types of psychiatric hospitalization offered for youth with eating disorders: specialized eating disorder units and general psychiatry units. The purpose of specialized eating disorder units is to provide ongoing support and management of eating disordered behaviors and cognitions, whereas the purpose of hospitalization of children with eating disorders on general child and adolescent inpatient units is for the management of significant comorbid psychiatry disorders or behavioral problems.

Specialized inpatient eating disorder program were common in the past; however, because of cost considerations and poor insurance coverage, many of these programs have closed and their function has been replaced by residential, day hospital or day treatment, and afterschool programs (see later discussion). In addition to the previously discussed programs, medically based programs focused on medical stability also serve some of the functions that previously were part of many specialized eating disorder inpatient programs. It is also noteworthy that in many part of the world outside the United States (eg, Japan, Germany, Singapore), such specialized inpatient programs are still a central element in treatments of children with eating disorders. Typically, these programs are behaviorally focused milieu headed by psychologists and psychiatrists, and supported by a team of specialized nurses, dieticians, social workers, and family therapists. The programmatic elements include structured meals, individual and group therapy, cognitive therapy, and family therapy, as well as many other supportive interventions, such as relaxation training, exercise training, and social skills groups. Most patients admitted to these types of services are underweight adolescents with anorexia nervosa, so the focus is on weight restoration. Lengths of stay vary widely from a few weeks to many months.

The rationale for the use of specialized inpatient eating disorder programs has been that professionals are better able than parents to help children with eating disorders disrupt maintaining behaviors such as severe dieting, overexercising, and purging. Although it is evident that these programs are often successful in accomplishing these goals, it is a challenge to translate these changes to the home setting. As a result, there is a high readmission rate after discharge. Data on the advantage of specialized inpatient eating disorder programs compared with outpatient interventions are highly limited; however, the available studies have not found an advantage overall for these specialty inpatient services compared with outpatient care. The first study to examine this question was published in 1991.[8] In that study, there were no differences in outcomes in those who received specialized inpatient eating disorder treatment compared with 3 types of outpatient regimens. The study included both adults and adolescents (average age of about 19 years) and was underpowered given the 4-cell design. Nonetheless, there was no indication of greater improvements on any outcome for the inpatient cohort. In a study of adolescents with anorexia nervosa specifically, Gowers and colleagues[9] again found no overall benefits to a specialized inpatient program compared with 2 outpatient regimens. This study was adequately powered; however, there were many participants who received treatments other than the treatment to which they were randomized. However, again, there were no differences between any of the groups except for cost. Hospitalization was by far the least cost-effective approach. These data do not suggest there is no role for specialized eating disorder inpatient programs for youth, who needs and will benefit from this high cost intervention remains unknown.

Inpatient psychiatric stays are appropriate when an individual is medically stable but is exhibiting behaviorally dangerous behaviors,such as uncontrolled binge eating, purging, or compulsive exercise. An advantage to this level of care is that length of stay does not depend solely on correcting medical abnormalities. Behavioral concerns are also taken into account when making a decision about when to discharge to the next level of care. Locked inpatient settings may be necessary for patients with active suicidal ideation or self-harming behaviors. It is particularly important for providers to assess safety regularly, given that approximately 50% of patients who succumb to eating disorders die by suicide.[2] Inpatient psychiatric units provide group therapy in addition to individual sessions with a therapist and psychiatrist. Psychopharmacological management may be necessary for patients with significant comorbid mood and anxiety concerns. Units typically have consulting pediatricians or family physicians on staff, can check laboratory and vital signs, and are usually able to use nasogastric tubes if needed. However, transition to a medical unit may be necessary should behaviors deteriorate to a point at which there is significant medical instability owing to acute food or fluid refusal.

Notably, not all general psychiatric units can adequately manage disordered eating behavior. Meal support and monitoring to prevent purging or overexercise is time and labor intensive, and requires that staff have special training to be alert to individuals who may be hiding or otherwise manipulating food. Some eating disorder treatment programs have specialized inpatient psychiatric units, other general programs have specialty eating disorder tracks embedded within the general program.

RESIDENTIAL TREATMENT CENTERS

The first residential eating disorder program opened in 1985, and by 2006, 22 programs were in operation. A survey at that time indicated that the average length of stay was 83 days, with an estimated daily cost of just under $1000 per day.[10] The number of programs and costs has only continued to escalate in the last 10-plus years, probably due to a decrease in inpatient hospitalization during the same period.[11] Residential treatment is typically indicated when a patient is medically and psychiatrically stable but still requiring more support than is possible at a lower level of care.[12] This may be due to difficult-to-manage urges to binge, purge, or exercise, or to chronic challenges regarding appropriate nutrition intake. Most eating disorder providers strongly prefer to keep young patients at home with their families if possible, given that it is disruptive and potentially traumatic to remove a young person from the comfort and safety of his or her home. However, adequate eating disorder treatment resources may not be locally available in all areas, and some patients require more support due to extreme disease severity, or because their family is struggling to implement treatment recommendations or does not agree with the philosophy of FBT.

Residential stays are generally 30, 60, 90, or more days, and require that the patient live in the treatment setting for this extended period of time. Residential facilities are typically more home-like than the hospital setting but are still staffed by nurses and milieu counselors. Patients have regular contact with medical providers and psychiatrists. They engage in regular group therapy sessions with peers, in addition to intensive individual and family therapy. Some programs focus on dialectical behavioral skills training, whereas others have a more cognitive behavioral therapy (CBT) philosophy. Still others use programming based on the principles of FBT. Patients are able to have therapeutic passes with families and staff for supervised therapeutic meal and snack challenges or clothing shopping excursions to target body image concerns. Many are located in geographic locations with mild weather and access to amenities such as massage therapy, hiking, art therapy, yoga, music, dance, and equestrian therapy. Decisions about discharge are often made based on an assessment of improvement in eating disorder thoughts and urges to engage in behaviors. Programs often recommend stepdown to day treatment, such as partial hospitalization programs (PHPs) or intensive outpatient programs (IOPs) that may be affiliated with the residential treatment center before full return to outpatient treatment.

PARTIAL HOSPITAL PROGRAMS

PHPs can be useful for patients who are struggling with structure and support at home but are medically and psychiatrically stable and want to have time at home with family in the evenings. When used as a stepdown, the time at home at night provides the patient with an opportunity to practice being more independent with nighttime snacks, as well as managing urges to engage in disordered eating behaviors for a short period of time during the day.[13]

PHPs vary in the length and frequency of expected attendance and participation. Most are open anywhere from 6 to 12 hours, Monday through Friday, although some are also open on weekends and holidays. They provide supervised meals and snacks, as well as group therapy, individual therapy, family sessions, and follow-up visits with medical and psychiatric providers. Different programs vary in their theoretic philosophy (CBT vs FBT) and may offer some of the amenities available in residential programs (eg, yoga, massage). Length of stay varies and can be anywhere from 2 weeks to 4 months, depending on progress. Many PHPs are also associated with IOPs, with overlap in programming. As with discharge from residential treatment, PHPs often recommend that the patient steps down to intensive outpatient treatment before a return to regular outpatient sessions.

INTENSIVE OUTPATIENT PROGRAMS

IOPs are similar to PHPs in that they provide meal support and a mix of group and individual therapy, along with medical and psychiatric follow-up. Some IOPs are free standing, whereas others are associated with PHPs. IOPs are typically 3 to 6 hours in duration and often run in the afternoon and evening hours so that patients may return to school and get practice managing eating behaviors and abstaining from binge or purge episodes and exercise, while also withstanding the associated academic and social stresses. The structure and support is also available during times when many feel particularly vulnerable to eating disorder behaviors. Typically, programs recommend that patients gradually taper the number of days that they attend each week in preparation for the transition to outpatient care. See **Table 2**.

EVIDENCE BASE

Although there is a lot of evidence to support the use of FBT in adolescent eating disorders,[18] outcomes data supporting higher levels of care are harder to come by. Medical and psychiatric inpatient stays are generally justified by the need to stabilize vital signs or to resolve a crisis situation. There is some evidence to suggest that patients who have been medically hospitalized for malnutrition tend to do better over the long

Table 2
Indications for higher levels of care in eating disorders

Inpatient Medical Hospitalization (see Table 1)	Inpatient Psychiatric Hospitalization (Medically Stable)	Residential Treatment Center (Medically and Psychiatrically Stable)	PHP (Medically and Psychiatrically Stable)	IOP (Medically and Psychiatrically Stable)
• Low weight (<75% median body mass index) • Unstable vital signs • Electrolyte abnormalities • Electrocardiogram abnormalities	• Acute suicidal ideation, recent suicide attempt, aborted suicide attempt • Acute food refusal • Uncontrolled binge eating, purging, exercise	• Needs professional supervision to eat regularly, gain weight, refrain from exercise and purging • 24 h, 7 d/wk	• Needs professional supervision and structure to eat regularly, gain weight, refrain from exercise and purging • ~8 h, 5–7 d/wk • Able to commute to program daily	• Increasingly self-sufficient to eat regularly, gain weight, refrain from exercise and purging • ~3–4 h, 2–5 d/wk • Able to commute to program daily

Data from Refs.[14–17]

term in terms of weight restoration, likely because the severity of medical illness helps both patient and parents take the situation more seriously than they might if the focus were entirely outpatient.[19] However, having required an inpatient medical hospitalization is also a predictor of poorer outcome in some outpatient treatments (eg, FBT and AFT).[20]

However, residential and PHP or IOP stays are often long, disruptive, and expensive. Some are not fully covered by insurance plans and require a substantial financial contribution from individuals and families. Some academic groups have recently voiced increasing concern about the marketing of for-profit programs, particularly because some of them have been criticized for being spa-like and offering activities that are not evidence-based alongside more traditional psychotherapy interventions. Many market directly to referring clinicians, and may offer meals, gifts, travel, and continuing medical education credits reminiscent of tactics used by the pharmaceutical industry in the past.[21] There has been a call for residential programs and PHPs or IOPs to increase transparency regarding outcomes measures by suggesting that all such programs submit outcomes data to an independent central entity so that patients and families can make an informed choice.[22]

The sparse literature available tends to provide demographic information about patients treated in these settings, and suggests that individuals restore weight and demonstrate improvement in eating disorder symptoms at discharge from the program, and at follow-up several years later.[23,24] A review of 25 open trials (19 PHPs and 6 residential programs) published between 2001 and 2015 reported improvement in weight and eating disorder behaviors at discharge, although follow-up data are spotty.[25] Further studies are needed to determine whether these improvements are sustained. One study suggested that extended inpatient hospitalization was not superior to short inpatient admission followed by a PHP for purposes of weight restoration.[26] However, there have not been any studies comparing PHPs or IOPs to outpatient care and, notably, many of these studies looked at adult populations rather than children and adolescents. Almost any structured treatment setting will help an individual achieve weight restoration over time. However, it is very common for patients to quickly default to preferred coping strategies such as restricting, binge eating, purging, and exercising when they return to the home environment. This frequently leads to weight loss, vital sign instability, and relapse back into the eating disorder. On the other hand, FBT encourages parents to provide oversight and accountability as the patient becomes more independent with eating and activity, and empowers them to step in to reverse relapsing behaviors quickly.

Clearly, more needs to be done to document the evidence to support higher levels of care, particularly given that they are extremely costly and progress may not be sustained as the patient transitions back to their regular environment. However, for patients and families in need of more support and structure than can be provided at home, higher levels of care can serve an important purpose in eating disorder treatment.

REFERENCES

1. Anderson LK, Reilly EE, Berner L, et al. Treating eating disorders at higher levels of care: overview and challenges. Curr Psychiatry Rep 2017;19:48.
2. Birmingham CS. The mortality rate from anorexia nervosa. Int J Eat Disord 2005; 38(2):143–6.
3. Golden N. Update on the medical management of eating disorders in adolescents. J Adolesc Health 2015;56(4):370–5.

4. Poulton A, Briody J, McCorquodale T, et al. Weight loss on stimulant medication: how does it affect body composition and bone metabolism?- A prospective longitudinal study. Int J Pediatr Endocrinol 2012;2012(1):30.

5. Golden N, Attia E. Psychopharmacology of eating disorders in children and adolescents. Pediatr Clin North Am 2011;58(1):121–38.

6. Goldstein DW, Wilson MG, Thompson VL, et al. Long term fluoxetine treatment of bulimia nervosa. Fluoxetine bulimia research group. Br J Psychiatry 1995;166(5): 660–6.

7. McElroy S, Hudson J, Mitchell J, et al. Efficacy and safety of lisdexamfetamine for treatment of adults with moderate to severe binge eating disorder: a randomized clinical trial. JAMA Psychiatry 2015;72(3):235–46.

8. Crisp AH, Norton K, Gowers S, et al. A controlled study of the effect of therapies aimed at adolescent and family psychopathology in anorexia nervosa. Br J Psychiatry 1991;159:325–33.

9. Gowers S, Clark A, Roberts C, et al. Clinical effectiveness of treatments for anorexia nervosa in adolescents. Br J Psychiatr 2007;191(5):427–35.

10. Frisch MJ, Herzog DB, Franko DL. Residential treatment for eating disorders. Int J Eat Disord 2006;39(5):434–42.

11. Zhao Y. An update on hospitalizations for eating disorders 199 to 2009, statistical brief #120, H-Cup healthcare cost and utilization project. Rockville (MD): Agency for Healthcare Research and Quality; 2001.

12. Fisher MM. Residential programs in the treatment of eating disorders. In: Fisher MM, Golden NG, editors. Adolescent medicine: state of the art reviews. Advances in adolescent eating disorders29. Itasca (IL): American Academy of Pediatrics; 2018. p. 404–12, 2.

13. Essayli JH, Ornstein RM. A review of partial hospitalization programs for the treatment of eating disorders in adolescents. In: Fisher MM, Golden NG, editors. Adolescent medicine: state of the art reviews. Advances in adolescent eating disorders29. Itasca (IL): American Academy of Pediatrics; 2018. p. 375–83, 2.

14. Lock J, LaVia M. Practice parameters for the assessment and treatment of children and adolescents with eating disorders. J Am Acad Child Adolesc Psychiatry 2015;54(5):412–25.

15. Golden N, Katzman D, Sawyer S, et al. Position Paper of the Society for Adolescent Health and Medicine: medical management of restrictive eating disorders in adolescents and young adults. J Adolesc Health 2015;56:121–5.

16. Yager J, Devlin M, Halmi K, et al. Practice guideline for the treatment of patients with eating disorders. 3rd edition. Washington, DC: American Psychiatric Association; 2006. p. 2012.

17. Rosen D, the Committee on Adolescence. Identification and management of eating disorders in children and adolescents. Pediatrics 2010;126(6):1240–53.

18. Lock J. An update on evidence-based psychosocial treatments for eating disorders in children and adolescents. J Clin Child Adolesc Psychol 2015;44(5): 707–21.

19. Kapphahn CJ, Graham DA, Woods ER, et al. Effect of hospitalization on percent median body mass index at one year, in underweight youth with restrictive eating disorders. J Adolesc Health 2017;61:310–6.

20. Peebles R, Hardy KK, Wilson JL, et al. Are diagnostic criteria for eating disorders markers of medical severity? Pediatrics 2010;125(5):e1193–201.

21. Attia E, Blackwood K, Guarda A, et al. Marketing residential treatment programs for eating disorders: a call for transparency. Psychiatr Serv 2016;67(6):664–6.

22. Attia E, Marcus M, Walsh BT, et al. The need for consistent outcome measures in eating disorder treatment programs: a proposal for the field. Int J Eat Disord 2017;50:231–4.
23. Brewerton T, Costin C. Long term outcome of residential treatment for anorexia nervosa and bulimia nervosa. Eat Disord 2011;19(2):132–44.
24. Brewerton T, Costin C. Treatment results of anorexia nervosa and bulimia nervosa in a residential treatment program. Eat Disord 2011;19(2):117–31.
25. Friedman K, Ramirez AL, Murray SB, et al. A narrative review of outcome studies for residential and partial hospital based treatment of eating disorders. Eur Eat Disord Rev 2016;24:263–76.
26. Herpertz-Dahlmann B, Schwarte R, Krei M, et al. Day-patient treatment after short inpatient care versus continued inpatient treatment in adolescents with anorexia nervosa (ANDI): a multicentre, randomised, open-label, non-inferiority trial. Lancet 2014;383:1222–9.

Psychotropic Medication for Children and Adolescents with Eating Disorders

Jennifer Couturier, MD, MSc[a],*, Leanna Isserlin, MD[b],
Wendy Spettigue, MD[b], Mark Norris, MD[b]

KEYWORDS

- Olanzapine • Risperidone • Selective serotonin reuptake inhibitors
- Anorexia nervosa • Bulimia nervosa • Avoidant restrictive food intake disorder

KEY POINTS

- Atypical antipsychotics are the most studied medications for children and adolescents with anorexia nervosa and have some evidence of efficacy, although studies are mixed.
- Selective serotonin reuptake inhibitors appear to have some usefulness in treating bulimia nervosa in children and adolescents, although results are very preliminary.
- More research is needed to determine which subgroups of young patients with eating disorders respond to each medication class.

INTRODUCTION

Despite advances in the number of medication-based studies completed in adolescent patients with eating disorders (EDs) over the last 2 decades, the field remains very much in its infancy. In contrast, emerging research suggests that psychotropic medications are used regularly in clinical care.[1–3] At present, 3 studies have examined the frequency of use of psychotropics in children and adolescents with EDs at the time of assessment and also at follow-up time points. Monge and colleagues[3] reported that at initial presentation 20.4% of 635 adolescents were taking psychotropic medication, and at 1-year follow-up, 58.7% were taking such medications. In this study, selective serotonin reuptake inhibitors (SSRIs) were the most commonly prescribed medications, and medication use was associated with a need for a higher level of care and psychiatric comorbidity (62.6%). More recently, Mizusaki and colleagues[2] reported that 45% of adolescents and young adults presenting to an academic EDs program

Disclosure Statement: The authors have no disclosures.
[a] McMaster University, McMaster Children's Hospital, 1200 Main Street West, Hamilton, Ontario L8N 3Z5, Canada; [b] University of Ottawa, Children's Hospital of Eastern Ontario, 401 Smyth Road, Ottawa, Ontario K1H 8L1, Canada
* Corresponding author.
E-mail address: coutur@mcmaster.ca

Child Adolesc Psychiatric Clin N Am 28 (2019) 583–592
https://doi.org/10.1016/j.chc.2019.05.005
1056-4993/19/© 2019 Elsevier Inc. All rights reserved.

childpsych.theclinics.com

were taking psychotropic medication. These investigators reported that only a minority of the patients in this sample had diagnosed comorbidity, and that diagnosis of Other Specified Eating Disorders, longer duration of illness, and a history of nonsuicidal self-injury increased the likelihood that a patient would be taking psychotropic medications. Finally, in a different sample, Garner and colleagues[1] reported that 80% of adolescents admitted to an ED residential program were taking psychotropic medication upon admission. Again, antidepressants were the most commonly prescribed medications.

Although by no means a complete picture, these studies provide insight into the prevalence at which medications are being used in this patient population and highlight the need for systematic reviews and clinical practice guidelines to be available to guide clinicians in their practice.

Only 1 North American guideline currently exists specifically focused on the treatment of children and adolescents with EDs.[4] To date, 3 systematic reviews have focused on medication treatments for EDs specifically in children and youth.[5–7] These reviews have suggested that the greatest body of evidence exists for olanzapine, with some studies showing positive effects on body mass index (BMI), ED symptoms, and function. However, significant limitations, including poor-quality study design, heterogeneity of assessment tools used, small sample sizes, and lack of adequate control groups, limit the ability of reviewers to draw definitive conclusions about the utility of olanzapine.[5]

This article reviews the literature on the efficacy of psychotropic medications used exclusively to treat children and adolescents with primary EDs. Systematic review methodology was used to capture all articles on psychopharmacology for EDs in children and adolescents. A search was performed in the following databases: PubMed, OVID, CIANHL, and Cochrane Database. The search terms "Anorexia Nervosa (AN)", "Bulimia Nervosa (BN)", "Binge Eating Disorder (BED)", "Other Specified Feeding and Eating Disorder (OSFED)", "Eating Disorder Not Otherwise Specified (EDNOS)", and "Avoidant/Restrictive Food Intake Disorder (ARFID)" were used, along with treatments such as Selective Serotonin Reuptake Inhibitors, Atypical Antipsychotics, Mood Stabilizers, and Serotonin Norepinephrine Reuptake Inhibitors. All articles up until November 2018 were reviewed. Reference lists were reviewed for any additional articles.

ANOREXIA NERVOSA
Atypical Antipsychotics

Olanzapine
Olanzapine has been the most commonly studied psychotropic medication for children and adolescents with anorexia nervosa (AN). At present, only 1 double-blind placebo-controlled trial in this population has been published. Kafantaris and colleagues[8] examined olanzapine in 20 underweight adolescents being treated in inpatient (n = 9), day treatment (n = 6), and outpatient (n = 5) settings (age range 12.3–21.8 years). In a 10-week pilot study, they found no differences in beneficial effect between the olanzapine and placebo groups in the 15 subjects who completed the trial; however, the treated group showed a trend toward increasing fasting glucose and insulin levels by the end of the study. The mean dose of olanzapine was 8.5 mg daily. Of note, only 21% of eligible patients were recruited into the study, and there was a high rate of attrition. Furthermore, patients were enrolled in each of inpatient, day hospital, and outpatient treatment setting as part of the study design. Although other research teams have also attempted randomized controlled trials using olanzapine in this population, trials have been hampered by a myriad of confounding and recruitment issues.[9]

Several open trials and case series have examined the use of olanzapine in children and adolescents with AN. The most recent of these studies enrolled 38 patients with AN, 22 of whom took olanzapine and 10 who declined medication and were retained as a comparison group. The mean dose of medication was 5.28 mg daily over a 12-week trial period. Those in the medication group demonstrated a significantly higher rate of weight gain in the first 4 weeks, although approximately one-third of participants discontinued olanzapine early due to side effects.[10]

Leggero and colleagues[11] reported a case series of 13 young patients (aged 9.6–16.3 years) treated with a mean dose of 4.13 mg daily of olanzapine. Significant improvements were seen in weight, functioning, ED symptoms, and hyperactivity. Similarly, Swenne and Rosling[12] reported 47 adolescents with AN treated with a mean dose of 5.1 mg daily. A mean weight gain of 9 kg was noted. The patients were treated for a mean of 228 days with olanzapine and were followed for 3 months following medication discontinuation. Biochemical side effects were closely monitored and were thought to be more related to refeeding processes than to medication.[12]

Hillebrand and colleagues[13] also reported olanzapine use in 7 patients (mean age 16.0 years) with AN. Most were taking 5 mg of olanzapine, with 1 patient receiving 15 mg once daily. The investigators found reductions in activity levels in the adolescents taking olanzapine in comparison to 11 adolescents not treated with olanzapine. All patients were receiving either inpatient or day hospital care, and there were no significant differences in weight.[13]

Norris and colleagues[14] completed a retrospective chart review of 22 inpatients treated with olanzapine compared with an untreated age-matched group. The rate of weight gain was not significantly different; however, the treated group had more psychiatric comorbidities than those not taking olanzapine and experienced side effects of sedation and dyslipidemia.[14]

Several smaller case series have also been published. Pisano and colleagues[15] report 5 cases of AN treated with 2.5 to 7.5 mg of olanzapine. At 6-month follow-up, these patients demonstrated increased oral intake and improved BMI. Dennis and colleagues[16] used olanzapine at a dose of 5 mg daily in 5 adolescent girls with AN and found an increase in BMI, reduction of body concerns, and improvements in sleep and anxiety surrounding food and weight. Another case series involving 4 young patients aged 10 to 12 years reported the use of olanzapine at a dose of 2.5 mg daily to treat AN.[17] These investigators reported improvements in compliance and weight gain as well as decreases in agitation. Mehler and colleagues[18] reported 5 female patients aged 12 to 17 years on a dose range of 5 mg to 12.5 mg daily of olanzapine. They found improvements in body image distortion and rigidity. La Via and colleagues[19] described 2 women with AN who experienced reduction of inner tension and "paranoid ideas" with use of 10 mg daily of olanzapine. Finally, there is a case report using olanzapine 5 mg daily to treat a 17-year-old girl with AN and comorbid pervasive developmental disorder not otherwise specified.[20] These investigators reported weight restoration and improvements in eating behavior within 5 months of initiating treatment.

Risperidone

Hagman and colleagues[21] conducted a double-blind placebo controlled trial of risperidone in adolescents and young adults with AN (age range 12–21 years). These investigators randomized 40 patients to risperidone or placebo. The mean dose of risperidone was 2.5 mg daily over a mean duration of 9 weeks. There were no differences found between the groups at the end of the study.[21] Personal communication with the primary investigator indicates that even when the subgroup of patients under the age of 18 years was examined, no differences were found. These investigators concluded that their results do not support the use of risperidone in the weight restoration phase of treatment of young patients with AN.[21]

The only other study found of the use of risperidone in the treatment of AN was a case report of a 12-year-old girl with autism and AN who was described as benefiting from treatment with risperidone at a dose of 0.5 mg twice daily.[22]

Quetiapine

Very few studies exist on the treatment of AN with quetiapine. One case series described quetiapine use in 3 subjects, aged 11 to 15 years with severe AN (lengthy hospitalization, use of nasogastric tubes, and BMI 12.3–13.9).[23] Two of these patients were treated with quetiapine 100 mg twice daily, and 1 patient was treated with 250 mg twice daily. Investigators reported improvements in body image disturbance, weight phobia, and "paranoid ideas." Sedation and constipation were noted as side effects. In a larger study also involving adults, Powers and colleagues[24] reported an open-label study of quetiapine. Six of the patients were adolescents aged 14 to 18 years in this study. The dose of quetiapine ranged from 150 mg daily to 300 mg daily. Improvements in anxiety and depression were noted, although the investigators report weight gain was modest at only 0.73 kg.[24]

Aripiprazole

Frank[25] completed a case series and a retrospective chart review[26] on the use of aripiprazole in adolescents with AN. The case series reported 4 adolescents who benefited in terms of weight and improved ED cognitions.[25] The chart review described 22 adolescents with AN taking aripiprazole at a mean dose of 3.59 mg daily compared with an untreated comparison group of 84 adolescents with AN. These investigators found a greater increase in BMI in the treated group.[26] One other case series reported the use of aripiprazole and included 1 adolescent with AN.[27] The adolescent received a dose of 5 mg daily. The investigators report an improvement in anxiety and rigidity around eating with aripiprazole.

Selective Serotonin Reuptake Inhibitors

There is 1 retrospective study comparing 19 adolescent patients with AN taking SSRIs with 13 patients with AN not treated with SSRIs.[28] These investigators found no differences between groups in terms of BMI, ED psychopathology, or depressive and obsessive-compulsive symptoms after evaluating patients on admission, discharge, and 1-year follow-up. The SSRIs involved in this study included fluoxetine (n = 7, mean dose 35 mg daily), fluvoxamine (n = 8, mean dose 120 mg daily), and sertraline (n = 4, mean dose 100 mg daily). One other case-control study examined fluoxetine as an adjunct to intensive multidisciplinary inpatient treatment.[29] No beneficial effect was found on global clinical severity of eating behavior or weight phobia. A case-control study by Wockel and colleagues[30] predominantly focused on the use of tricyclic antidepressants in 25 adolescents with AN; however, fluvoxamine was also used in 2 of the subjects. Those patients who had comorbid depression seemed to have a more robust platelet serotonin-receptor calcium release in response to antidepressants.[30] Three adolescent case reports have been published on the use of SSRIs in AN. One on the use of sertraline in an adolescent with AN with symptoms of purging[31]; another on the use of fluoxetine in an adolescent with AN and depressive features,[32] and another on the use of fluoxetine for comorbid obsessive compulsive disorder.[33] All of these cases described a benefit in terms of anxiety, mood, and weight restoration.

Other Antidepressants

Mirtazapine

To date, 1 case control study as well as 2 case reports involving the use of mirtazapine in AN have been published. Hrdlicka and colleagues[34] examined 9 adolescent patients with AN who had been treated with mirtazapine for anxiety or depression compared with 9 female controls with AN. The 2 groups were matched in terms of age and BMI. The mean dose of mirtazapine was 21.7 mg daily. There were no significant differences in terms of weight or BMI at the end of this study.[34] The first case report described a 16-year-old girl hospitalized for AN and depression treated with mirtazapine.[35] These investigators found positive results in terms of weight restoration and mood improvement and suggested further study of the medication was needed. More recently, Naguy and Al-Mutairi[36] described the case of a 16-year-old boy hospitalized for severe AN who responded well to mirtazapine 30 mg/d in terms of weight restoration.

Combinations of Medications

Other case reports have focused on a combination of treatments with antipsychotics and antidepressants, which makes interpretation of the results difficult. For example, Newman-Toker[37] describes 2 cases of adolescents with AN in which risperidone (1.5 mg daily) was added to antidepressant treatment, with improvements in anxiety and weight gain. Similarly, Ercan and colleagues[38] described a case of a 15-year-old girl with severe AN treated with olanzapine, fluoxetine, alprazolam, and thioridazine, demonstrating that polypharmacy is sometimes needed for severe symptoms of AN, including agitation and fear of weight gain. These investigators also reported that once stabilized in terms of agitation, a maintenance dose of 10 mg of olanzapine daily resulted in an increase in BMI, along with a reduction of obsessive-compulsive symptoms, exercising, and anorexic cognitions in this patient.[38]

BULIMIA NERVOSA

Selective Serotonin Reuptake Inhibitors

SSRIs have shown the most promise for children and youth with bulimia nervosa (BN), although the evidence is scant. One open trial of fluoxetine in 10 adolescents aged 12 to 18 years[39] reported 8 weeks of a titrating dose of fluoxetine (maximum 60 mg daily) along with supportive psychotherapy. Frequencies of binge episodes decreased significantly from a mean of 4.1 to 0 episodes per week, and weekly purges decreased from 6.4 to 0.4 episodes.[39] Seventy percent of patients were rated as improved or much improved on the clinical global impressions-improvement scale. No significant side effects were noted. Whether patients maintained these benefits over the long term is unknown.

Other Psychotropic Medications

One case report describes the use of valproate 200 mg twice daily following onset of mania thought to be related to the use of fluoxetine in an adolescent girl with BN. In this report, mood stabilized and binge-eating and purging symptoms resolved once the fluoxetine had been stopped and valproate was initiated.[40]

Finally, 1 paper described the use of stimulants to treat BN with comorbid attention-deficit/hyperactivity disorder (ADHD).[41] The 2 cases of adolescents treated with dextroamphetamine 5 to 10 mg 3 times daily had a rapid response to the medication, including improved concentration and no further binge or purge episodes.

BINGE-EATING DISORDER

No studies could be located that specifically address psychopharmacologic treatment of binge-eating disorder in children and adolescents. Lisdexamfetamine has been approved by the Food and Drug Administration for binge-eating disorder in adults, but has not been studied in child and adolescent populations.

AVOIDANT/RESTRICTIVE FOOD INTAKE DISORDER

Avoidant/restrictive food intake disorder (ARFID) is a heterogeneous diagnostic category often associated with multiple underlying causes for food restriction. In a recent case series, Spettigue and colleagues[42] described 6 patients with ARFID and comorbid anxiety (median age 12.9 years) who were treated with a combination of family therapy plus pharmacotherapy. All patients were treated with olanzapine in combination with other medications, making interpretation of the results difficult: 3 cases were treated with a combination of olanzapine and fluoxetine; 1 case was treated with olanzapine followed by fluvoxamine, and 2 cases were treated with a combination of olanzapine, cyproheptadine, and fluoxetine. All 6 cases reached their treatment goal weights. Of note, this is the only report in the literature of cyproheptadine for the treatment of ARFID.

Another recent case series reported beneficial effects from olanzapine in the treatment of patients with ARFID.[43] These investigators completed a retrospective chart review and described a significant increase in weight as well as improvements in anxiety and depressive symptoms in 9 patients with ARFID treated with olanzapine. The mean final dose of olanzapine was 2.8 mg daily. All 9 patients had comorbid mental health diagnoses, including separation anxiety, obsessive-compulsive disorder, posttraumatic stress disorder, generalized anxiety disorder, and social anxiety disorder. Six of the 9 also had significant major depressive symptoms.

In terms of the "posttraumatic" subtype of ARFID whereby there has been a choking event followed by refusal to eat and drink, several medications have been described in case reports as being helpful, including lorazepam,[44] mirtazapine,[45] escitalopram,[46] and fluoxetine.[47] Of note, Celik and colleagues[47] reported a case of two 2-year old twins who were treated with fluoxetine 5 mg daily for severe posttraumatic food avoidance, with good effect. Similarly, a case series of 3 children with "severe choking phobias" were successfully treated with low-dose SSRIs (sertraline and paroxetine),[48] and a case report described the beneficial use of fluoxetine (20 mg daily) in combination with aripiprazole (2.5 mg daily) for a 15-year-old girl with severe choking phobia.[49]

Pennell and colleagues[50] described 2 cases whereby significant weight loss occurred with stimulant treatment of ADHD, resulting in the need for hospitalization. These cases were managed by temporarily stopping the stimulant and adding risperidone to help with appetite and behavior.

An additional case report describes a 15-year-old girl with anxiety, somatic symptoms of nausea, and abdominal pain who benefited from treatment with buspirone 7.5 mg twice daily after becoming agitated with a course of sertraline.[51]

OTHER SPECIFIED FEEDING AND EATING DISORDERS

The authors' review identified 1 case report of a patient with atypical AN whose depressive symptoms were treated with escitalopram with improvement noted.[52] She had lost almost 40 kg over a period of 4 months, but remained within a normal weight range.

LACK OF EVIDENCE

No studies could be found on the use of selective norepinephrine reuptake inhibitors for this population. The same was true for mood stabilizers. The only reports found for benzodiazepines are mentioned above for ARFID and in the combination of treatments with other medications for AN.

SUMMARY

Most of the published studies to date on pharmacotherapy of EDs in children and adolescents have focused on the role of antipsychotic medication in AN. Despite progress in recent years, the total number of subjects studied remains small, and there is a paucity of randomized controlled trials. Furthermore, it has become increasingly clear that there are substantive challenges involved with the completion of such studies. As a result, there is still insufficient evidence to recommend medication as a first-line consideration in children and adolescents with EDs. Because of the significant challenges in recruitment and retention in clinical trials to date, large multisite collaborative trials are necessary to move the field forward in determining which young patients with EDs might benefit most from psychotropic medication and in what fashion.

REFERENCES

1. Garner DM, Anderson ML, Keiper CD, et al. Psychotropic medications in adult and adolescent eating disorders: clinical practice versus evidence-based recommendations. Eat Weight Disord 2016;21(3):395–402.
2. Mizusaki K, Gih D, LaRosa C, et al. Psychotropic usage by patients presenting to an academic eating disorders program. Eat Weight Disord 2018. https://doi.org/10.1007/s40519-018-0520-3.
3. Monge MC, Forman SF, McKenzie NM, et al. Use of psychopharmacologic medications in adolescents with restrictive eating disorders: analysis of data from the National Eating Disorder Quality Improvement Collaborative. J Adolesc Health 2015;57(1):66–72.
4. Lock J, La Via MC, American Academy of Child and Adolescent Psychiatry (AACAP) Committee on Quality Issues (CQI). Practice parameter for the assessment and treatment of children and adolescents with eating disorders. J Am Acad Child Adolesc Psychiatry 2015;54(5):412–25.
5. Balestrieri M, Oriani MG, Simoncini A, et al. Psychotropic drug treatment in anorexia nervosa. Search for differences in efficacy/tolerability between adolescent and mixed-age population. Eur Eat Disord Rev 2013;21(5):361–73.
6. Couturier J, Lock J. A review of medication use for children and adolescents with eating disorders. J Can Acad Child Adolesc Psychiatry 2007;16(4):173–6.
7. van den Heuvel LL, Jordaan GP. The psychopharmacological management of eating disorders in children and adolescents. J Child Adolesc Ment Health 2014;26(2):125–37.
8. Kafantaris V, Leigh E, Hertz S, et al. A placebo-controlled pilot study of adjunctive olanzapine for adolescents with anorexia nervosa. J Child Adolesc Psychopharmacol 2011;21(3):207–12.
9. Norris ML, Spettigue W, Buchholz A, et al. Factors influencing research drug trials in adolescents with anorexia nervosa. Eat Disord 2010;18(3):210–7.
10. Spettigue W, Norris ML, Maras D, et al. Evaluation of the effectiveness and safety of olanzapine as an adjunctive treatment for anorexia nervosa in adolescents: an open-label trial. J Can Acad Child Adolesc Psychiatry 2018;27(3):197–208.

11. Leggero C, Masi G, Brunori E, et al. Low-dose olanzapine monotherapy in girls with anorexia nervosa, restricting subtype: focus on hyperactivity. J Child Adolesc Psychopharmacol 2010;20(2):127–33.

12. Swenne I, Rosling A. No unexpected adverse events and biochemical side effects of olanzapine as adjunct treatment in adolescent girls with eating disorders. J Child Adolesc Psychopharmacol 2011;21(3):221–7.

13. Hillebrand JJ, van Elburg AA, Kas MJ, et al. Olanzapine reduces physical activity in rats exposed to activity-based anorexia: possible implications for treatment of anorexia nervosa? Biol Psychiatry 2005;58(8):651–7.

14. Norris ML, Spettigue W, Buchholz A, et al. Olanzapine use for the adjunctive treatment of adolescents with anorexia nervosa. J Child Adolesc Psychopharmacol 2011;21(3):213–20.

15. Pisano S, Catone G, Pascotto A, et al. Second generation antipsychotics in adolescent anorexia nervosa: a new hypothesis of eligibility criteria. J Child Adolesc Psychopharmacol 2014;24(5):293–5.

16. Dennis K, Le Grange D, Bremer J. Olanzapine use in adolescent anorexia nervosa. Eat Weight Disord 2006;11(2):e53–6.

17. Boachie A, Goldfield GS, Spettigue W. Olanzapine use as an adjunctive treatment for hospitalized children with anorexia nervosa: case reports. Int J Eat Disord 2003;33(1):98–103.

18. Mehler C, Wewetzer C, Schulze U, et al. Olanzapine in children and adolescents with chronic anorexia nervosa. A study of five cases. Eur Child Adolesc Psychiatry 2001;10(2):151–7.

19. La Via MC, Gray N, Kaye WH. Case reports of olanzapine treatment of anorexia nervosa. Int J Eat Disord 2000;27(3):363–6.

20. Tateno M, Teshirogi H, Kamasaki H, et al. Successful olanzapine treatment of anorexia nervosa in a girl with pervasive developmental disorder not otherwise specified. Psychiatry Clin Neurosci 2008;62(6):752.

21. Hagman J, Gralla J, Sigel E, et al. A double-blind, placebo-controlled study of risperidone for the treatment of adolescents and young adults with anorexia nervosa: a pilot study. J Am Acad Child Adolesc Psychiatry 2011;50(9):915–24.

22. Fisman S, Steele M, Short J, et al. Case study: anorexia nervosa and autistic disorder in an adolescent girl. J Am Acad Child Adolesc Psychiatry 1996;35(7):937–40.

23. Mehler-Wex C, Romanos M, Kirchheiner J, et al. Atypical antipsychotics in severe anorexia nervosa in children and adolescents—review and case reports. Eur Eat Disord Rev 2008;16(2). https://doi.org/10.1002/erv.843.

24. Powers PS, Bannon Y, Eubanks R, et al. Quetiapine in anorexia nervosa patients: an open label outpatient pilot study. Int J Eat Disord 2007;40(1):21–6.

25. Frank GK. Aripiprazole, a partial dopamine agonist to improve adolescent anorexia nervosa—a case series. Int J Eat Disord 2016;49(5):529–33.

26. Frank GK, Shott ME, Hagman JO, et al. The partial dopamine D2 receptor agonist aripiprazole is associated with weight gain in adolescent anorexia nervosa. Int J Eat Disord 2017;50(4):447–50.

27. Trunko ME, Schwartz TA, Duvvuri V, et al. Aripiprazole in anorexia nervosa and low-weight bulimia nervosa: case reports. Int J Eat Disord 2011;44(3):269–75.

28. Holtkamp K, Konrad K, Kaiser N, et al. A retrospective study of SSRI treatment in adolescent anorexia nervosa: insufficient evidence for efficacy. J Psychiatr Res 2005;39(3):303–10.

29. Strober M, Pataki C, Freeman R, et al. No effect of adjunctive fluoxetine on eating behavior or weight phobia during the inpatient treatment of anorexia nervosa: an

historical case-control study. J Child Adolesc Psychopharmacol 1999;9(3): 195–201.

30. Wockel L, Koch S, Stadler C, et al. Serotonin-induced platelet intracellular Ca2+ response in patients with anorexia nervosa. Pharmacopsychiatry 2008; 41(1):10–6.

31. Frank GK, Kaye WH, Marcus MD. Sertraline in underweight binge eating/purging-type eating disorders: five case reports. Int J Eat Disord 2001;29(4):495–8.

32. Lyles B, Sarkis E, Kemph JP. Fluoxetine and anorexia. J Am Acad Child Adolesc Psychiatry 1990;29(6):984–5.

33. Gee RL, Telew N. Obsessive-compulsive disorder and anorexia nervosa in a high school athlete: a case report. J Athl Train 1999;34(4):375–8.

34. Hrdlicka M, Beranova I, Zamecnikova R, et al. Mirtazapine in the treatment of adolescent anorexia nervosa. Case-control study. Eur Child Adolesc Psychiatry 2008;17(3):187–9.

35. Jaafar NR, Daud TI, Rahman FN, et al. Mirtazapine for anorexia nervosa with depression. Aust N Z J Psychiatry 2007;41(9):768–9.

36. Naguy A, Al-Mutairi A. An adolescent male with anorexia nervosa favorably responded to mirtazapine. Am J Ther 2018;25(6):e675–6.

37. Newman-Toker J. Risperidone in anorexia nervosa. J Am Acad Child Adolesc Psychiatry 2000;39(8):941–2.

38. Ercan ES, Copkunol H, Cykoethlu S, et al. Olanzapine treatment of an adolescent girl with anorexia nervosa. Hum Psychopharmacol 2003;18(5):401–3.

39. Kotler LA, Devlin MJ, Davies M, et al. An open trial of fluoxetine for adolescents with bulimia nervosa. J Child Adolesc Psychopharmacol 2003;13(3):329–35.

40. Tor PC, Lee EL. Treatment emergent mania responding to valproate in a Chinese female adolescent population with eating disorders: a case series. Eur Eat Disord Rev 2008;16(6):421–6.

41. Dukarm CP. Bulimia nervosa and attention deficit hyperactivity disorder: a possible role for stimulant medication. J Womens Health (Larchmt) 2005;14(4): 345–50.

42. Spettigue W, Norris ML, Santos A, et al. Treatment of children and adolescents with avoidant/restrictive food intake disorder: a case series examining the feasibility of family therapy and adjunctive treatments. J Eat Disord 2018;6:20.

43. Brewerton TD, D'Agostino M. Adjunctive use of olanzapine in the treatment of avoidant restrictive food intake disorder in children and adolescents in an eating disorders program. J Child Adolesc Psychopharmacol 2017;27(10):920–2.

44. Kardas M, Cermik BB, Ekmekci S, et al. Lorazepam in the treatment of posttraumatic feeding disorder. J Child Adolesc Psychopharmacol 2014;24(5):296–7.

45. Tanidir C, Herguner S. Mirtazapine for choking phobia: report of a pediatric case. J Child Adolesc Psychopharmacol 2015;25(8):659–60.

46. Hosoglu E, Akca OF. Escitalopram in the treatment of a 3-year-old child with posttraumatic feeding disorder. J Child Adolesc Psychopharmacol 2018;28(2):153–4.

47. Celik G, Diler RS, Tahiroglu AY, et al. Fluoxetine in posttraumatic eating disorder in two-year-old twins. J Child Adolesc Psychopharmacol 2007;17(2):233–6.

48. Banerjee SP, Bhandari RP, Rosenberg DR. Use of low-dose selective serotonin reuptake inhibitors for severe, refractory choking phobia in childhood. J Dev Behav Pediatr 2005;26(2):123–7.

49. Colak Sivri R, Hizarcioglu Gulsen H, Yilmaz A. Phagophobia successfully treated with low-dose aripiprazole in an adolescent: a case report. Clin Neuropharmacol 2018;41(4):148–50.

50. Pennell A, Couturier J, Grant C, et al. Severe avoidant/restrictive food intake disorder and coexisting stimulant treated attention deficit hyperactivity disorder. Int J Eat Disord 2016;49(11):1036–9.

51. Okereke NK. Buspirone treatment of anxiety in an adolescent female with avoidant/restrictive food intake disorder. J Child Adolesc Psychopharmacol 2018; 28(6):425–6.

52. Wolter H, Schneider N, Pfeiffer E, et al. Diagnostic crossover from obesity to atypical anorexia nervosa—a case report. Obes Facts 2009;2(1):52–3.

Medical Complications of Eating Disorders in Youth

Rebecka Peebles, MD[a],*, Erin Hayley Sieke, MD, MS[b]

KEYWORDS

- Medical complications • Malnutrition • Weight restoration

KEY POINTS

- It is important that medical providers screen for eating disorders. Dieting, overexercise, or a recent drop in weight may indicate the need for a more thorough work-up.
- Bias can cause clinicians to miss evidence of disordered eating in higher-weight patients, leading to potentially serious delays in appropriate care.
- It is important to diagnose eating disorders accurately and involve families in education and treatment.
- Eating disorders can cause problematic medical complications in every organ system.

INTRODUCTION

Eating disorders (EDs) affect more than 30 million Americans and many more youth worldwide.[1] EDs are varied and include binge-eating disorder as most prevalent but also bulimia nervosa (BN) and anorexia nervosa (AN), avoidant-restrictive food intake disorder, purging disorder, atypical AN, and others.[2,3] EDs do not discriminate: youth of all genders, sizes, ethnicities, and socioeconomic strata can develop these life-threatening illnesses.[4–11] EDs can cause tremendous emotional suffering and significant medical consequences and have up to a 10% mortality rate.[12,13] With early and appropriate intervention, most medical complications can be recognized and reversed, although many sufferers do not access care and, therefore, can go on to develop chronic sequelae. Because of this, helping identify, refer, and treat youth with EDs to get effective care is critical to their future emotional and physical recovery.[14]

Disclosure Statement: The authors have nothing to disclose. Dr R. Peebles' work is supported by the National Institutes of Health (K23DK100558), and the Hilda and Preston Davis Foundation.
[a] Eating Disorder Assessment and Treatment Program, The Children's Hospital of Philadelphia, Perelman School of Medicine at The University of Pennsylvania, Roberts Center for Pediatric Research, 2716 South Street, Room 14360, Philadelphia, PA 19146, USA; [b] The Children's Hospital of Philadelphia, 3401 Civic Center Boulevard 9NW55, Philadelphia, PA 19104, USA
* Corresponding author.
E-mail address: peeblesr@email.chop.edu

EDs in youth can have an impact on every organ system, and complications can occur at any weight. Providers must be alert to potential complications, particularly in youth with EDs, who can often present in an atypical fashion.[15,16] This review delineates medical presentations and complications of EDs in youth by organ system rather than by diagnosis, because EDs can exist on a spectrum and share many physiologic similarities. Emphasis is placed on the pediatric literature, but when medical sequelae of EDs are not well described in youth, studies of adult populations may be referenced.

GENERAL MEDICAL APPROACH

Since the recent adaptation of behavioral criteria into the diagnostic criteria in the *Diagnostic and Statistical Manual of Mental Disorders* (Fifth Edition), there has been greater recognition that children and adolescents with EDs may not verbalize abstract concepts, such as fear of weight gain or overt body distortions. Complicating diagnosis further, these youth may not lose dramatic weight but may simply not grow appropriately over time, and linear growth stunting is not always quickly recognized.[17] Finally, many medical providers continue to carry long-held biases that prevent them from identifying EDs in young children, males, youth of color, and youth of normal or higher weights. It is important to be aware that EDs are more common than type 2 diabetes mellitus in youth and work to recognize these illnesses in all patients, even those who may not present in a stereotypical fashion.[14,18,19]

An ED should be suspected in a patient of any weight who presents with weight loss, unexplained growth stunting or pubertal delay, restrictive or abnormal eating behaviors, recurrent vomiting, excessive exercise, trouble gaining weight, or body image concerns. Screening for dieting, excessive exercise, and concerns about weight is helpful in identifying some high-risk youth. Growth trajectories and body mass index (BMI) curves should be assessed at each visit; if drops in percentiles are noted, the child should be screened further to assess if there are any concerning behaviors that led to this change.[14,18,19] Given newer data implicating drops in growth curve percentiles as being putative risk identifiers of future EDs,[20] it is prudent to counsel caregivers of the importance of keeping growth on target during the pediatric years, with extra attention to adequate nutrition to allow for normal individual trajectories. BMI suppression, or the difference between patients' highest BMI percentile and their percentile at presentation for treatment of their ED, should be noted, because reducing weight suppression is important in reversing many medical complications.[21–26] When an ED is suspected, a comprehensive history and physical examination (**Box 1**) can help support next steps. Remembering to obtain ancillary history from caregivers is important, because many youth with EDs may not be forthcoming about specific behaviors of concern. An appropriate differential diagnosis (**Box 2**) should be considered during the evaluation, and laboratory testing (**Box 3**) can help to detect complications as well as possible causes of the malnutrition and dysregulated eating behaviors noted on examination.[18]

EATING DISORDERS IN LARGER BODIES

Youth of all sizes can suffer from disordered eating, and a subset of larger-bodied youth is vulnerable to AN, BN, and other EDs. Medical providers frequently are more practiced in screening for lipid abnormalities and insulin resistance than for disordered eating behaviors in patients of higher weights. They also can be biased toward only looking for eating disorders in thin patients, which can often can lead to dangerous delays in care. If emerging AN is missed in a higher-weight patient who

---

Box 1
History and physical examination considerations

Features to ask about on history (note: gather history from both patient and a caregiver because some reports may vary considerably if behaviors are secretive)

- Onset/duration of symptoms and any previous treatment/attempts at treatment
- Weight trajectory—highest and lowest weights and time course (obtain lifetime growth curves if at all possible)
- Maladaptive weight control behaviors: purging, binge eating, fasting, diet pills, diuretics, and laxative use (both prescribed and nonprescribed)
- Special diets: vegan/vegetarian, low-carbohydrate/low-fat/paleo/ketogenic
- Food phobias or aversions, including textural aversions
- Swallowing or choking fears/sensations
- 24-hour food recall
- Exercise history—current activity as well as typical activity if patient's activity has been modified lately, secretive exercise, exercise when sick/injured, and driven/compulsive quality to exercise
- Menstrual history if female
- Fracture history
- Careful past medical, social (do not forget self-harm, mood changes, bullying, trauma, substance use or abuse, and high-risk behaviors), and family history (in particular, history of gastrointestinal conditions, including celiac disease and inflammatory bowel disorders, sudden cardiac events, inflammatory disease, cystic fibrosis, anxiety/obsessive compulsive disorder, suicide or depression, EDs or difficulty, and substance abuse)
- Medications, including supplements and over-the-counter medications
- Review of symptoms: cold intolerance, poor circulation, chest pain, syncope, headaches, constipation or diarrhea, abdominal pain, reflux, nonvolitional vomiting, sleep difficulties, mood changes, hair loss, and weakness

Physical examination findings of note

- Abnormalities in vital signs (bradycardia, hypotension, and hypothermia)
- Acrocyanosis, cold distal extremities
- Russell sign—callous or marking over finger(s) induced by repetitive vomiting
- Lanugo—fine downy hair
- Yellow/orange skin discoloration—indicative of excessive carotene consumption in setting of high intake of carotenoids
- Self-harm scars
- Parotid gland enlargement—if bilateral, nontender, noninflamed, and symmetric, can be due to purging
- Gag reflex—can be absent in chronic purging
- Tooth enamel erosions
- Tanner staging to assess pubertal stage; can note breast tissue atrophy as well
- Edema

Box 2
Differential diagnosis of poor growth/weight gain, hypogonadism, or recurrent vomiting/binge eating in youth

- Gastrointestinal disease: celiac disease, Crohn disease, ulcerative colitis, gastroparesis, eosinophilic esophagitis/gastroenteritis, superior mesenteric artery syndrome, median arcuate ligament syndrome, liver disease, gastroesophageal reflux, and pancreatitis

- Endocrine disease: thyroid disorders, diabetes, pregnancy, prolactinomas, Addison disease, growth hormone deficiency, congenital adrenal hyperplasia, and polycystic ovarian syndrome

- Oncologic causes: consider brain tumors, leukemia, lymphoma, and bone marrow dyscrasias

- Inflammatory/rheumatologic conditions: juvenile rheumatoid arthritis, Raynaud syndrome, and systemic lupus erythematosus

- Genetic: Prader-Willi syndrome and Turner syndrome

- Postural orthostatic tachycardia syndrome

- Renal failure

- Neurologic conditions: autism spectrum disorders, neurodegenerative disorders, and abdominal migraine

- Psychological conditions: depression, bipolar disease, anxiety disorders, and psychotropic medication side effects (depressed appetite or growth on medications for attention deficit disorder, increased appetite on neuroleptics or atypical antipsychotics)

- Vitamin deficiencies: vitamin B_{12}, thiamine, zinc, iron, and vitamin D

- Less common: porphyria, human immunodeficiency virus, tuberculosis, and mast cell activation syndrome

Note: these illnesses can also coexist with an eating disorder; thus, diagnosis of an organic cause of poor growth or weight gain does not rule out the presence of a comorbid ED

---

is embarking on weight loss in an unsafe manner, critical windows for early intervention are missed. Instead, often an ED is caught when it has become far too entrenched, after many providers have congratulated the patient on weight loss in the meantime. It is important to remember that weight loss is difficult to accomplish, and that, when consistent and rapid weight loss is seen over time, EDs always should be screened for and it should be ensured that there are no extreme weight control behaviors emerging, even if the young person is not an abnormally low weight on a growth chart. Research has shown that patients who are higher weight but have a clinical ED can still experience life-threatening complications.[14,27,28]

INVOLVING FAMILIES

Medical providers often are the first professionals to diagnose an ED in children, and the interactions surrounding this first encounter can reverberate over time. EDs used to be thought of as chronic diseases, and afflicted youth were not thought likely to fully recover. Because effective interventions that allowed long-term recovery did not exist, medical providers hesitated to name these disorders in pediatric patients, because the diagnosis itself often felt hopeless. It is now well-established that many cognitions and complications of EDs can fully reverse with appropriate weight restoration and interruption of the ED behaviors. Caregivers and parents have proved in multiple studies to be effective and essential partners in the treatment process. Therefore, providers

---

Box 3
Laboratory testing for initial evaluation of youth with suspected eating disorders

- Complete blood cell count
- Comprehensive metabolic profile, including phosphorus and magnesium levels
- Thyroid function testing
- Erythrocyte sedimentation rate (if high normal or high, consider inflammatory conditions on differential)
- Amylase and lipase
- Prolactin
- Vitamin D, ferritin, thiamine; consider vitamin B_{12} (best test is methylmalonic acid level) and zinc as well, particularly if strict vegan or vegetarian diet
- Male patients: total testosterone, FSH, and LH
- Female patients: estradiol, FSH, LH, and urine pregnancy test
- Electrocardiogram
- Consider celiac disease screen if high-risk family history or symptoms (total IgA level, antitissue transglutaminase IgA, and antiendomysial antibody IgA)
- If short stature: consider Insulin-like Growth Factor 1 (IGF-1) and Insulin-like Growth Factor Binding Protein 3 (IGF-BP3)
- If significant vomiting or abdominal pain: upper gastrointestinal series with small bowel follow-through or gastric emptying study may be useful
- If significant neurologic findings or concerns: brain magnetic resonance imaging may be useful
- If significant hypogonadism on testing, or greater than 6 months amenorrhea for female patients, OR multiple long bone or stress fractures, consider DXA testing to assess bone density—only worth obtaining at a pediatric center with good technique and established track record of accurate testing and interpretation in youth

---

should be straightforward about their concerns with both patients and parents early in the evaluation process and should work in a similarly upfront manner to alleviate stigma associated with the diagnosis of an ED by explaining how common they are and how effective treatment can be.[29]

CARDIOVASCULAR COMPLICATIONS

Cardiac complications are common and are associated with one-third of the deaths in ED patients.[30–32] Evaluating heart rate and blood pressure both supine and standing and obtaining an electrocardiogram are standard in the baseline cardiovascular assessment of the eating disordered adolescent. Up to 80% of adolescent patients with AN present with some cardiac complication, such as bradycardia and hypotension, rhythm abnormalities, and changes in heart rate variability and autonomic function.[33] Physical symptoms may vary but can include dizziness, syncope, palpitations, and headache, although many patients remain asymptomatic even in the presence of significant vital sign instability.[34]

Many patients with restrictive EDs have significantly decreased left ventricular mass, decreased cardiac output, and decreased stroke volume on echocardiogram.[35,36] Cardiac mass often is decreased in weight loss,[37] and this can lead to systolic dysfunction and low heart rates, because the heart tries to make adaptive changes to lower its workload. The cardiac muscle achieves this by reducing cardiac output and slowing the heart rate. Several additional mechanisms have been proposed for bradycardia in AN and include an increase in vagal tone and decreased metabolic rate.[36] Vagal tone has also been noted to be increased in adult bulimic women engaging in some caloric restriction.[38] Bradycardia is commonly reported in children with all types of EDs at presentation.[27]

Although uncommon, QTc prolongation has been noted in a small percentage of children with EDs at presentation. In a case-control study of outpatient adolescents with AN, 40% had QTc intervals greater than 440 ms, whereas none of the controls presented with any prolongation.[37] Another study showed that the largest predictor of QTc interval dispersion, defined as the range between shortest and longest QTc intervals, was weight loss.[39] Some studies have suggested that purging may play a role in QTc prolongation, with BN patients demonstrating significantly longer QTc intervals than patients with AN.[27] These findings highlight the importance of checking an electrocardiogram on all patients with EDs, regardless of weight, because patients with BN tend to be in a normal weight range.

Nearly one-third of hospitalized patients with AN have mitral valve prolapse and pericardial effusions.[33,40–43] Several small studies have demonstrated almost complete reversibility of both structural and functional derangement,[42,43] although ipecac abuse in patients who purge can lead to an irreversible cardiomyopathy.[44–48] These cardiovascular complications can occur in patients of all weights, particularly if they have recently lost weight or engaged in restrictive or purging behaviors.[27,38,49–54]

ENDOCRINE DISTURBANCES AT PRESENTATION

Multiple endocrine abnormalities have been identified in adolescents with EDs, and these abnormalities, such as amenorrhea, pubertal delay, growth stunting, infertility, or changes in mood,[55–59] may be what drives patients and their families to seek care. It is imperative that medical providers prioritize obtaining a thorough menstrual and/or pubertal history, accurate height and growth trajectories, Tanner staging, and obtaining baseline laboratory testing assessing luteinizing hormone (LH), follicle-stimulating hormone (FSH), estradiol, and, in cases of men, testosterone levels in assessing any possible endocrine disruptions that have occurred due to an ED.[14]

Decreased energy availability, stress, sleep abnormalities, fat mass loss, and excessive exercise can all contribute to hypothalamic hypogonadotropic hypogonadism in youth with EDs.[56,60–62] Manifestations of this include pubertal delay or regression, primary or secondary amenorrhea in female youth, and decreased nocturnal emissions or morning erections in male youth.[55–59,63] In a study of adolescents, 28% of 11 year olds to 18 year olds with AN had primary amenorrhea compared with 11% of normal-weight adolescents.[64] Amenorrhea also has been described in up to 40% of BN subjects and 34% of eating disorder not otherwise specified subjects.[65] Although female youth with EDs often present with suppressed gonadotropins and estradiol levels, studies of male youth with AN also have demonstrated lower gonadotropin and testosterone levels.[66–69]

BN also is associated with a significantly greater level of hirsutism and polycystic ovarian syndrome and lower levels of FSH, LH, and estrogen.[70–74] Vomiting may have a direct but yet unknown effect on the hypothalamic pituitary axis: in a large sample of 2791 high school girls, those who reported binge eating 1 time to 3 times a month were 1.6 times more likely to have irregular menses, and those who purged more than once a week were 3 times as likely to have irregular menses.[75]

Menstrual function and gonadotropin levels typically recover after patients reach a healthy weight.[76,77] There is no agreed-on weight cutpoint that determines return of pubertal function for male youth and female youth; more recent studies indicate that recovering weight to a point that weight suppression is minimized for each individual is more important than achieving a specific percentile marker on a growth curve.[78,79] This means that patients in larger bodies may need to achieve a goal weight above the median for their age, if they have always been at a higher weight pre-ED, because this is what lessens their weight suppression and allows their endocrine system to repair.

Growth retardation in early adolescents with EDs is a significant problem clinically and likely results from growth hormone resistance and decreased insulinlike growth factor 1 (IGF-1) concentrations. Although premenarchal females and males with AN in either early puberty or midpuberty can achieve significant growth with weight gain and pubertal resumption, many still do not reach their target (midparental) height and have height deficits that persist. These findings emphasize the importance of weight restoration and treatment during adolescence, because continued weight loss may result in severe growth retardation.[61,80,81]

EDs also can result in low IGF-1, low to low-normal thyroxine and triiodothyronine levels, and sick euthyroid syndrome.[82] These abnormalities frequently resolve with weight restoration to a nonmalnourished state. ED adolescents also risk reduced bone mineral density primarily due to poor nutritional intake, low BMI, and reduced fat mass.[55,56,58,64,83–87] Leptin plays a key role in energy homeostasis, and levels are low in malnourished states.[55,60,88–92] Recent studies demonstrate that if leptin levels are normalized, menstrual function and thyroid and bone markers improve in hypothalamic amenorrhea.[93–96]

METABOLIC RATE AND RESTING ENERGY EXPENDITURE IN EATING DISORDERS

Alterations in resting metabolic rate are observed during both the starvation and refeeding phases of AN and other restrictive EDs.[97–101] Studies of metabolic rate during the acute starvation phase in AN have demonstrated resting metabolic rates that are 49% to 91% of predicted values.[98–101] The etiology of reduced metabolic rate in AN is multifactorial. First and foremost, metabolic rate is closely related to both total body mass and lean mass, and AN is characterized by significantly low body weight, leading to decreased lean mass. Thus, decreases in lean mass in AN lead to significant reductions in metabolic activity due to the decline in metabolically active tissue.[56,97] Other contributors to suppression of metabolic rate in AN may include suppression of thyroid hormone triiodothyronine and thyroxine[56,61] and decreased levels of circulating leptin. Lowered metabolic rates also have been documented in patients with BN with similar contributors.[100,102]

As patients are refed and weight restored, metabolic rate increases rapidly and substantially. With this increase in metabolic rate, the caloric intake needed to continue weight restoration correspondingly increases, contributing to the difficulty of achieving weight restoration. These changes in metabolic rate are explained only partially by the increase in total body mass and lean mass observed during refeeding.[103,104] Multiple studies have demonstrated substantial increases in resting metabolic rate during refeeding that could not be explained by weight gain, plasma norepinephrine, or thyroid hormones.[105] Impairments in nutrient digestion, absorption, transport, and storage; alterations in gut microbiota; low efficiency of lean tissue of storage; and alterations in diet induced thermogenesis have been hypothesized to be contributors to the complex disturbances of energy metabolism during refeeding in AN. Patients with anorexia may have caloric requirements that are 3 times their predicted resting energy requirements in order to achieve appropriate weight gain goals during recovery.[106]

HEMATOLOGIC ABNORMALITIES

Patients with EDs, in particular those with low BMIs, have been noted to have bone marrow hypoplasia and even gelatinous bone marrow transformation in some cases, which may result in leukopenia, anemia, and/or thrombocytopenia.[64,107–112] Neutropenia and lymphopenia also have been described and may increase the risk of infection in patients.[113,114] These abnormalities are all reversible with appropriate weight gain. Therefore, although vitamin B_{12} and iron studies may be prudent when cytopenias occur, bone marrow biopsies usually are deferred until after weight restoration is progressing well and only if the cytopenias persist.[115,116] Malnourished patients also typically have a low sedimentation rate, usually below 5 mm/h.[117,118] If the sedimentation rate is significantly elevated, inflammatory conditions should be considered in the differential diagnosis.

NEUROCOGNITIVE COMPLICATIONS

Malnutrition has multiple impacts on the growing brain in children and adolescents with EDs. Patients with severe AN have reduced brain tissue volume and impaired neurocognitive function on examination. Some studies have demonstrated persistent gray-white matter deficits on MRI even after weight restoration, but these findings are mixed in the literature and it is unclear how permanent structural and functional brain changes are in youth with EDs.[119–125] Similarly, studies on neurocognitive function have shown varied results.[126–140] Abnormalities in brain structure have been associated with low body weight and cortisol levels, whereas cognitive deficits are associated with menstrual function.[141]

Another neurocognitive complication of EDs involves anosognosia. This term was first developed to describe patients who, after having strokes, still believed that certain limbs would work and move when they clearly did not. It is now a term used in the field of EDs that has replaced earlier, more pejorative terms, like denial, because it reflects the fact that most patients feel fine even when they are medically and psychiatrically impaired.[142,143] Anosognosia is a hallmark of many EDs and, although it does typically resolve with treatment, it makes the initial stages of care more challenging because it is hard to convince patients that they require intervention.

GASTROINTESTINAL DISTURBANCES

Malnutrition, vomiting, and binge eating all can result in gastrointestinal complications. Delayed gastric emptying, manifesting in constipation, bloating, fullness, reflux, and abdominal pain, is common in EDs, although it has been better studied in adults than youth. Patients who vomit can have increased salivary amylase production, enlarged parotid glands, esophageal tears, and hematemesis and rarely can experience esophageal rupture and/or pneumomediastinum.[144–151] EDs also rarely can result in pancreatitis or liver disease, with typically mild elevations in pancreatic or hepatic enzymes.[152–156] Hyperlipidemia also is common but typically resolves with weight restoration.[157–161] Superior mesenteric artery syndrome is a well-described complication that can occur after significant weight loss; in this serious condition, the vascular supply to the small intestine can be disrupted and patients experience significant abdominal pain, particularly with meals, that is often out of proportion to physical exam findings.[86,153,162] Patients with binge-eating behaviors are at additional risk for gastric dilation or rarely gastric rupture and pancreatitis.[163–174]

COMPLICATIONS OF THE RENAL SYSTEM

Youth with EDs frequently develop dehydration and renal insufficiency due to severe fluid restriction or vomiting. Other renal abnormalities at presentation can include pyuria and, less commonly, proteinuria and hematuria, which both clear with hydration and reversal of malnutrition.[82] Patients with AN may lose renal concentrating ability, which can result in high urine output and inaccurate specific gravity measurements on urinalyses as well as excessive urine losses.[175–178]

ELECTROLYTE DISTURBANCES

Electrolyte disturbances can result from restricted dietary intake, vomiting, laxative abuse, or diuretic use and can be life-threatening. The most common electrolyte abnormalities seen are hypokalemia and hypophosphatemia. Hypochloremic metabolic alkalosis may develop in patients who vomit frequently, and hyperchloremic metabolic acidosis may develop in those who abuse laxatives. Patients with malnutrition are at risk for refeeding syndrome during treatment, which includes hypophosphatemia, hypokalemia, and hypomagnesemia.[179–189]

Because these complications often reflect more chronic, serious depletions, malnutrition does not always result in abnormal laboratory values, and normal laboratory values should not be taken as a measure of stability. Some electrolyte disturbances arise after the onset of refeeding, and, therefore, special attention should be paid to laboratory results during this time. The refeeding process can bring about a shift in metabolism as the body begins to metabolize glucose.[188,190–195] Phosphorous, magnesium, and potassium are the electrolytes that are most involved in this metabolic change, and, therefore, hypophosphatemia, hypokalemia, and hypomagnesmia are the most common electrolyte abnormalities.[196,197] In a study of severely malnourished adolescents with AN, 75% of the patients had a phosphorous nadir during the first week of refeeding.[187] Phosphorous levels should be closely monitored during hospitalization, because adverse effects of hypophosphatemia include cardiac failure, immune dysfunction, and death.[198] Careful, monitored refeeding and phosphorous supplementation can help mitigate the risk of refeeding syndrome.[187]

Other less common electrolyte and laboratory value abnormalities are hyponatremia, hypochloremia, and hypoglycemia. Hyponatremia may develop if patients with EDs drink excessive amounts of water before medical appointments in order to appear heavier[199] but is cause for concern due to the potential of seizures.[200,201] A study of AN and BN adult women reported hypochloremia prevalence of 8.1% but found that hypochloremia was most common in patients with frequent purging episodes.[183] Hypoglycemia is also rare but significant in AN. Severe hypoglycemia has been noted in several case reports of adults and may contribute to syncope, dissociative episodes, and potentially hypoglycemic coma.[202–206] In general, further studies need to be conducted on the effects of disordered eating behaviors on electrolyte and laboratory abnormalities in adolescents.

VITAMIN AND MICRONUTRIENT DISTURBANCES

Vitamin and mineral deficiencies are common in youth with EDs. The most common complications noted in the literature are vitamin D, calcium, and iron deficiencies, although thiamine and zinc deficiencies also are well described. These disturbances may contribute to ED symptoms, such as fatigue, decreased bone mass, depression, and reduced taste.[207-211]

TREATMENT CONSIDERATIONS IN YOUTH WITH EATING DISORDERS

Medical providers must become adept at working with a multidisciplinary team in managing youth with EDs. The role of the medical provider remains to ensure medical safety and resumption of normal physiologic and pubertal processes, with reversal or minimization of as many complications as possible. Ideally, if a youth is involved in appropriate therapy with an experienced practitioner or team, decisions about activity and calories should not be made in the medical office, other than just to determine the safety of the options being discussed. Because changes to activity and calories often involve behavioral stability even more than medical, parents and therapists should be heavily involved, if not driving, these decisions. If dieticians are involved, they also indicate basic safety guidelines and suggestions but let the parents and therapist make the final decisions. In this way, parents can help continue to implement the work at home with confidence and knowledge that they have been a part of the decision making throughout. Typically, all adolescents should be followed frequently throughout care for markers of pubertal development and physiologic stability, as previously outlined, and patients who purge should be even more closely followed due to their higher risk of electrolyte instability and QTc prolongation.

CRITERIA FOR EMERGENCY MEDICAL HOSPITALIZATION FOR ADOLESCENTS WITH EATING DISORDERS

Although most youth with EDs are safely managed as outpatients, the severity of some medical complications can warrant hospitalization. The Society for Adolescent Health and Medicine and the American Academy of Pediatrics have published consensus-derived criteria for medical stabilization, determined specifically for children and adolescents, as adapted in **Box 4**.[14,18,19,34,212] Findings consistent with these criteria support the decision to medically admit a patient for initiation of nutrition and stabilization. The degree of malnutrition is assessed in several ways, as evidenced in **Box 5**[212,213]; meeting any of these criteria indicates significant malnutrition. Malnutrition does not always mandate a low weight but also can be found when a young person experiences significant weight loss from a higher weight or does not gain expected weight over time. Many hospitals are moving toward more aggressive nutritional protocols because multiple studies have documented increased lengths of stay with no additional benefit using older paradigms of start low, go slow that advocate lower calories advanced over much longer periods of time. Some have shown promising outcomes after discharge in continued rates of weight gain at home.[14,18,19,34,106,212-216]

SUPPORTING OPTIMAL WEIGHT RESTORATION AND RECOVERY

Although there is no one agreed-on metric for recovery, most investigators agree that normalizing eating patterns, weight restoration, and the return of cognitive flexibility around eating all are important components. In addition, improved and age-appropriate functioning in psychological and social domains is considered critical. Weight and body shape should not drive maladaptive decision making, and normal growth, pubertal, and physiologic patterns should resume. To achieve recovery, adequate weight restoration typically is critical to the process.

Box 4
Typical criteria supportive of inpatient medical stabilization of youth with eating disorders

- BMI: <75% median BMI for age and gender by Centers for Disease Control and Prevention growth curves (https://www.cdc.gov/growthcharts/cdc_charts.htm)

- Heart rate: <50 beats per minute during day

- Systolic blood pressure: <90 mm Hg

- Temperature: <36.3°C

- Orthostasis: pulse increase >20 or systolic blood pressure decrease >10 mm Hg from lying (5 min) to standing (2 min)

- Hematemesis

- Syncope

- Arrhythmia or QT/QTc prolongation

- Electrolyte disturbances (eg, hypophosphatemia, hyponatremia, hypoglycemia, hypomagnesemia, and hypokalemia)

- Acute medical complications of malnutrition (seizures, cardiac failure, pancreatitis, renal failure, etc.)

- Significant psychiatric comorbidities, making outpatient management inappropriate

- Acute, significant food refusal that threatens hydration or health

Adapted from Golden NH, Katzman DK, Kreipe RE, et al. Eating disorders in adolescents: position paper of the Society for Adolescent Medicine. J Adolesc Health 2003;33(6):497; and Rosen DS. Identification and management of eating disorders in children and adolescents. Pediatrics 2010;126(6):1248; with permission.

A healthy weight is different from person to person. More centers are advocating that children and adolescents have goal weights set that are congruent with their lifetime, pre-ED growth trajectories to reduce BMI suppression and improve long-term outcomes. Thus, pediatric patients need to initially catch up weight so that their weight, height, and BMI curves return to their own individual trajectory, and then they need to continue growing as other children their age, on their growth curves, should grow. There is no such thing as a maintenance weight in youth, and this is important to emphasize in medical visits. Youth continue to grow and develop into young adulthood; even when they are done growing linearly, they should be adding bone mass, lean body mass, fat mass, and organ mass—and all of these contribute to the need for continued weight gain.

To determine an initial goal weight, consulting with a dietician may be helpful. Factors, such as midparental height, as well as birth weight and birth history often are useful in assessing if the young person was growing well before the ED started. Examining prior BMI growth curves can be helpful to help aim for patients to return to their preillness growth patterns. Patients who have arrested linear growth prior to presentation due to their low weight frequently need to weigh more than their natural BMI curve in order to kick-start and catch up height.

If no prior growth curves are available, a median body weight based on the 50th percentile BMI for age may be a starting point. Some patients, however, are most healthy above the median and some below the median. There is no one number that works for everyone and weight is considered along with other metrics of recovery to determine with the entire treatment team when weight restoration is truly complete. Emphasizing to parents and adolescents that goal weights are moving targets

---

Box 5
Considerations in grading severity of malnutrition

Mild malnutrition
- 80% to 90% median BMI for age/gender
- BMI z score: -1.0 to -1.99
- Weight loss: >10% preillness weight
- Deceleration in BMI across 1 z score or Centers for Disease Control and Prevention growth curve line
- Eating 51% to 75% of estimated needs

Moderate malnutrition
- 70% to 79% median BMI for age/gender
- BMI z score: -2.0 to -2.99
- Weight loss: >15% preillness weight
- Deceleration in BMI across 2 z score or Centers for Disease Control and Prevention growth curve lines
- Eating 26% to 50% of estimated needs

Severe malnutrition
- Less than 70% median BMI for age/gender
- BMI z score: ≤-3.0
- Weight loss: >20% preillness weight in 1 year or >10% in 6 months
- Deceleration in BMI across 3 z score or Centers for Disease Control and Prevention growth curve lines
- Eating $\leq$25% of estimated needs

Note: linear growth stunting as noted on growth curves could indicate severe malnutrition.

Adapted from Society for Adolescent Health and Medicine, Golden NH, Katzman DK, et al. Position paper of the Society for Adolescent Health and Medicine: medical management of restrictive eating disorders in adolescents and young adults. J Adolesc Health 2015;56(1):123; and Becker P, Carney LN, Corkins MR, et al. Consensus Statement of the Academy of Nutrition and Dietetics/American Society for Parenteral and Enteral Nutrition: Indicators Recommended for the Identification and Documentation of Pediatric Malnutrition (Undernutrition). Nutr Clin Pract 2015;30(1):158; with permission.

---

throughout adolescence can be helpful as a reminder that normal teens continue to grow throughout that time, and thus patients recovering from EDs also should continue to grow and gain as they get older.[14,19,29,106,215,217]

NUTRITIONAL NEEDS

Most pediatric patients with EDs require high calorie levels in treatment and for up to 2 years after reaching recovery. Calorie needs of 3000 kcal to 6000 kcal daily are not unusual, because patients with EDs can be hypermetabolic as a result of the metabolic consequences of malnutrition and refeeding. It is important not to reduce calorie levels prematurely and to normalize the amounts required so that families can adjust. As activity levels increase, calorie levels may need to increase as well rather than decrease later in treatment.[14,19,106,212–215,218,219]

SUMMARY

Children and adolescents with EDs of all genders and sizes are at risk of myriad medical disturbances due to their illness. These complications can be severe and life threatening and can have an impact on every organ system. The majority can be partially or fully reversed, however, with adequate treatment that attends to adequate weight restoration and cessation of maladaptive eating behaviors. Treatment may involve inpatient medical stabilization when necessary but always involves adequate nutrition. Involving caregivers in treatment has greatly improved outcomes. Advances in understanding the need for sufficient calories and weight restoration continue to unfold but indicate that many patients require far more calories and weight gain than previously thought to optimize their long-term recovery. Increased research in this field likely will elucidate important considerations for treatment. Ultimately, the severity of the medical consequences emphasizes the need for early identification and interdisciplinary treatment.

REFERENCES

1. Eating Disorder Coalition. Eating disorders: what the research shows 2016. Available at: http://eatingdisorderscoalition.org.s208556.gridserver.com/couch/uploads/file/fact-sheet_2016.pdf. Accessed July 16, 2019.
2. Hudson JI, Hiripi E, Pope HG Jr, et al. The prevalence and correlates of eating disorders in the National Comorbidity Survey Replication. Biol Psychiatry 2007; 61(3):348–58.
3. Le Grange D, Swanson SA, Crow SJ, et al. Eating disorder not otherwise specified presentation in the US population. Int J Eat Disord 2012;45(5):711–8.
4. Murray SB, Nagata JM, Griffiths S, et al. The enigma of male eating disorders: a critical review and synthesis. Clin Psychol Rev 2017;57:1–11.
5. Limbers CA, Cohen LA, Gray BA. Eating disorders in adolescent and young adult males: prevalence, diagnosis, and treatment strategies. Adolesc Health Med Ther 2018;9:111–6.
6. Mancini G, Biolcati R, Pupi V, et al. Eating disorders in males: an overview of research over the period 2007-2017. Riv Psichiatr 2018;53(4):177–91.
7. Pinhas L, Morris A, Crosby RD, et al. Incidence and age-specific presentation of restrictive eating disorders in children: a Canadian Paediatric Surveillance Program study. Arch Pediatr Adolesc Med 2011;165(10):895–9.
8. Becker CB, Middlemass K, Taylor B, et al. Food insecurity and eating disorder pathology. Int J Eat Disord 2017;50(9):1031–40.
9. Udo T, Grilo CM. Prevalence and correlates of DSM-5-defined eating disorders in a nationally representative sample of U.S. adults. Biol Psychiatry 2018;84(5): 345–54.
10. Calzo JP, Blashill AJ, Brown TA, et al. Eating disorders and disordered weight and shape control behaviors in sexual minority populations. Curr Psychiatry Rep 2017;19(8):49.
11. Rodrigues M. Do hispanic girls develop eating disorders? A critical review of the literature. Hisp Health Care Int 2017;15(4):189–96.
12. Arcelus J, Mitchell AJ, Wales J, et al. Mortality rates in patients with anorexia nervosa and other eating disorders. A meta-analysis of 36 studies. Arch Gen Psychiatry 2011;68(7):724–31.
13. Sullivan PF. Mortality in anorexia nervosa. Am J Psychiatry 1995;152:1073–4.
14. Campbell K, Peebles R. Eating disorders in children and adolescents: state of the art review. Pediatrics 2014;134(3):582–92.
15. Atkins DM, Silber TJ. Clinical spectrum of anorexia nervosa in children. J Dev Behav Pediatr 1993;14(4):211–6.
16. Bryant-Waugh R, Lask B. Eating disorders in children. J Child Psychol Psychiatry 1995;36(2):191–202.

17. Peebles R, Wilson JL, Lock JD. How do children with eating disorders differ from adolescents with eating disorders at initial evaluation? J Adolesc Health 2006; 39(6):800–5.
18. Golden NH, Katzman DK, Kreipe RE, et al. Eating disorders in adolescents: position paper of the Society for Adolescent Medicine. J Adolesc Health 2003; 33(6):496–503.
19. Golden NH, Katzman DK, Sawyer SM, et al. Update on the medical management of eating disorders in adolescents. J Adolesc Health 2015;56(4):370–5.
20. Yilmaz Z, Gottfredson NC, Zerwas SC, et al. Developmental premorbid body mass index trajectories of adolescents with eating disorders in a longitudinal population cohort. J Am Acad Child Adolesc Psychiatry 2019;58(2):191–9.
21. Accurso EC, Lebow J, Murray SB, et al. The relation of weight suppression and BMIz to bulimic symptoms in youth with bulimia nervosa. J Eat Disord 2016;4:21.
22. Berner LA, Shaw JA, Witt AA, et al. The relation of weight suppression and body mass index to symptomatology and treatment response in anorexia nervosa. J Abnorm Psychol 2013;122(3):694–708.
23. Bodell LP, Keel PK. Weight suppression in bulimia nervosa: associations with biology and behavior. J Abnorm Psychol 2015;124(4):994–1002.
24. Bodell LP, Racine SE, Wildes JE. Examining weight suppression as a predictor of eating disorder symptom trajectories in anorexia nervosa. Int J Eat Disord 2016;49(8):753–63.
25. Butryn ML, Lowe MR, Safer DL, et al. Weight suppression is a robust predictor of outcome in the cognitive-behavioral treatment of bulimia nervosa. J Abnorm Psychol 2006;115(1):62–7.
26. Lowe MR, Berner LA, Swanson SA, et al. Weight suppression predicts time to remission from bulimia nervosa. J Consult Clin Psychol 2011;79(6):772–6.
27. Peebles R, Hardy KK, Wilson JL, et al. Are diagnostic criteria for eating disorders markers of medical severity? Pediatrics 2010;125(5):e1193–201.
28. Whitelaw M, Gilbertson H, Lee KJ, et al. Restrictive eating disorders among adolescent inpatients. Pediatrics 2014;134(3):e758–64.
29. Katzman DK, Peebles R, Sawyer SM, et al. The role of the pediatrician in family-based treatment for adolescent eating disorders: opportunities and challenges. J Adolesc Health 2013;53(4):433–40.
30. Sharp CW, Freeman CP. The medical complications of anorexia nervosa. Br J Psychiatry 1993;162:452–62.
31. Isner JM, Roberts WC, Heymsfield SB, et al. Anorexia nervosa and sudden death. Ann Intern Med 1985;102(1):49–52.
32. Neumarker KJ. Mortality and sudden death in anorexia nervosa. Int J Eat Disord 1997;21(3):205–12.
33. Olivares JL, Vazquez M, Fleta J, et al. Cardiac findings in adolescents with anorexia nervosa at diagnosis and after weight restoration. Eur J Pediatr 2005;164(6):383–6.
34. Rosen DS. Identification and management of eating disorders in children and adolescents. Pediatrics 2010;126(6):1240–53.
35. Galetta F, Franzoni F, Cupisti A, et al. Early detection of cardiac dysfunction in patients with anorexia nervosa by tissue Doppler imaging. Int J Cardiol 2005; 101(1):33–7.
36. Galetta F, Franzoni F, Prattichizzo F, et al. Heart rate variability and left ventricular diastolic function in anorexia nervosa. J Adolesc Health 2003;32(6):416–21.
37. Vazquez M, Olivares JL, Fleta J, et al. Cardiac disorders in young women with anorexia nervosa. Rev Esp Cardiol 2003;56(7):669–73 [in Spanish].

38. Vogele C, Hilbert A, Tuschen-Caffier B. Dietary restriction, cardiac autonomic regulation and stress reactivity in bulimic women. Physiol Behav 2009;98(1–2):229–34.
39. Swenne I, Larsson PT. Heart risk associated with weight loss in anorexia nervosa and eating disorders: risk factors for QTc interval prolongation and dispersion. Acta Paediatr 1999;88(3):304–9.
40. Kastner S, Salbach-Andrae H, Renneberg B, et al. Echocardiographic findings in adolescents with anorexia nervosa at beginning of treatment and after weight recovery. Eur Child Adolesc Psychiatry 2012;21(1):15–21.
41. Katzman DK. Medical complications in adolescents with anorexia nervosa: a review of the literature. Int J Eat Disord 2005;37(Suppl):S52–9 [discussion S87–59].
42. Mont L, Castro J, Herreros B, et al. Reversibility of cardiac abnormalities in adolescents with anorexia nervosa after weight recovery. J Am Acad Child Adolesc Psychiatry 2003;42(7):808–13.
43. Oflaz S, Yucel B, Oz F, et al. Assessment of myocardial damage by cardiac MRI in patients with anorexia nervosa. Int J Eat Disord 2013;46(8):862–6.
44. Effects of ipecac on the heart. N Engl J Med 1986;314(19):1253–5.
45. Birmingham CL, Gritzner S. Heart failure in anorexia nervosa: case report and review of the literature. Eat Weight Disord 2007;12(1):e7–10.
46. Brotman MC, Forbath N, Garfinkel PE, et al. Myopathy due to ipecac syrup poisoning in a patient with anorexia nervosa. Can Med Assoc J 1981;125(5):453–4.
47. Friedman EJ. Death from ipecac intoxication in a patient with anorexia nervosa. Am J Psychiatry 1984;141(5):702–3.
48. Ho PC, Dweik R, Cohen MC. Rapidly reversible cardiomyopathy associated with chronic ipecac ingestion. Clin Cardiol 1998;21(10):780–3.
49. Brown CA, Mehler PS. Medical complications of self-induced vomiting. Eat Disord 2013;21(4):287–94.
50. Buchanan R, Ngwira J, Amsha K. Prolonged QT interval in bulimia nervosa. BMJ Case Rep 2011;2011 [pii:bcr0120113780].
51. Kennedy SH, Heslegrave RJ. Cardiac regulation in bulimia nervosa. J Psychiatr Res 1989;23(3–4):267–73.
52. Messerli-Burgy N, Engesser C, Lemmenmeier E, et al. Cardiovascular stress reactivity and recovery in bulimia nervosa and binge eating disorder. Int J Psychophysiol 2010;78(2):163–8.
53. Nahshoni E, Yaroslavsky A, Varticovschi P, et al. Alterations in QT dispersion in the surface electrocardiogram of female adolescent inpatients diagnosed with bulimia nervosa. Compr Psychiatry 2010;51(4):406–11.
54. Takimoto Y, Yoshiuchi K, Kumano H, et al. Bulimia nervosa and abnormal cardiac repolarization. J Psychosom Res 2006;60(1):105–7.
55. Baskaran C, Misra M, Klibanski A. Effects of anorexia nervosa on the endocrine system. Pediatr Endocrinol Rev 2017;14(3):302–11.
56. Misra M, Klibanski A. Endocrine consequences of anorexia nervosa. Lancet Diabetes Endocrinol 2014;2(7):581–92.
57. Mitchell JE, Bantle JP. Metabolic and endocrine investigations in women of normal weight with the bulimia syndrome. Biol Psychiatry 1983;18(3):355–65.
58. Munoz MT, Argente J. Anorexia nervosa in female adolescents: endocrine and bone mineral density disturbances. Eur J Endocrinol 2002;147(3):275–86.
59. Russell GF. Clinical and endocrine features of anorexia nervosa. Trans Med Soc Lond 1971;87:40–50.
60. Ahima RS. Body fat, leptin, and hypothalamic amenorrhea. N Engl J Med 2004;351(10):959–62.

61. Misra M, Klibanski A. Neuroendocrine consequences of anorexia nervosa in adolescents. Endocr Dev 2010;17:197–214.
62. Boyar RM, Katz J, Finkelstein JW, et al. Anorexia nervosa. Immaturity of the 24-hour luteinizing hormone secretory pattern. N Engl J Med 1974;291(17):861–5.
63. Skolnick A, Schulman RC, Galindo RJ, et al. The endocrinopathies of male anorexia nervosa: case series. AACE Clin Case Rep 2016;2(4):e351–7.
64. Misra M, Aggarwal A, Miller KK, et al. Effects of anorexia nervosa on clinical, hematologic, biochemical, and bone density parameters in community-dwelling adolescent girls. Pediatrics 2004;114(6):1574–83.
65. Poyastro Pinheiro A, Thornton LM, Plotonicov KH, et al. Patterns of menstrual disturbance in eating disorders. Int J Eat Disord 2007;40(5):424–34.
66. Toifl K, Waldhauser F, Lischka A, et al. Anorexia nervosa in male adolescents. II. Psychoneuroendocrinologic findings. Klin Padiatr 1988;200(4):316–20 [in German].
67. Tomova A, Kumanov F, Andreeva M. Endocrine changes in males with anorexia nervosa: 2 of the authors' own cases. Vutr Boles 1991;30(1):48–53 [in Bulgarian].
68. Tomova A, Kumanov P. Sex differences and similarities of hormonal alterations in patients with anorexia nervosa. Andrologia 1999;31(3):143–7.
69. Misra M, Katzman DK, Cord J, et al. Bone metabolism in adolescent boys with anorexia nervosa. J Clin Endocrinol Metab 2008;93(8):3029–36.
70. Naessen S, Carlstrom K, Garoff L, et al. Polycystic ovary syndrome in bulimic women–an evaluation based on the new diagnostic criteria. Gynecol Endocrinol 2006;22(7):388–94.
71. Resch M, Szendei G, Haasz P. Bulimia from a gynecological view: hormonal changes. J Obstet Gynaecol 2004;24(8):907–10.
72. Morgan JF, McCluskey SE, Brunton JN, et al. Polycystic ovarian morphology and bulimia nervosa: a 9-year follow-up study. Fertil Steril 2002;77(5):928–31.
73. Morgan JF. Polycystic ovary syndrome, gestational diabetes, and bulimia nervosa. J Clin Endocrinol Metab 1999;84(12):4746.
74. Raphael FJ, Rodin DA, Peattie A, et al. Ovarian morphology and insulin sensitivity in women with bulimia nervosa. Clin Endocrinol 1995;43(4):451–5.
75. Austin SB, Ziyadeh NJ, Vohra S, et al. Irregular menses linked to vomiting in a nonclinical sample: findings from the National Eating Disorders Screening Program in high schools. J Adolesc Health 2008;42(5):450–7.
76. Golden NH, Jacobson MS, Schebendach J, et al. Resumption of menses in anorexia nervosa. Arch Pediatr Adolesc Med 1997;151(1):16–21.
77. Faust JP, Goldschmidt AB, Anderson KE, et al. Resumption of menses in anorexia nervosa during a course of family-based treatment. J Eat Disord 2013;1:12.
78. Seetharaman S, Golden NH, Halpern-Felsher B, et al. Effect of a prior history of overweight on return of menses in adolescents with eating disorders. J Adolesc Health 2017;60(4):469–71.
79. Dempfle A, Herpertz-Dahlmann B, Timmesfeld N, et al. Predictors of the resumption of menses in adolescent anorexia nervosa. BMC Psychiatry 2013;13:308.
80. Lantzouni E, Frank GR, Golden NH, et al. Reversibility of growth stunting in early onset anorexia nervosa: a prospective study. J Adolesc Health 2002;31(2):162–5.
81. Modan-Moses D, Yaroslavsky A, Novikov I, et al. Stunting of growth as a major feature of anorexia nervosa in male adolescents. Pediatrics 2003;111(2):270–6.

82. Palla B, Litt IF. Medical complications of eating disorders in adolescents. Pediatrics 1988;81(5):613–23.
83. Douyon L, Schteingart DE. Effect of obesity and starvation on thyroid hormone, growth hormone, and cortisol secretion. Endocrinol Metab Clin North Am 2002; 31(1):173–89.
84. Gianotti L, Lanfranco F, Ramunni J, et al. GH/IGF-I axis in anorexia nervosa. Eat Weight Disord 2002;7(2):94–105.
85. Legroux-Gerot I, Vignau J, D'Herbomez M, et al. Evaluation of bone loss and its mechanisms in anorexia nervosa. Calcif Tissue Int 2007;81(3):174–82.
86. Mehler PS, Brown C. Anorexia nervosa - medical complications. J Eat Disord 2015;3:11.
87. Reinehr T, Isa A, de Sousa G, et al. Thyroid hormones and their relation to weight status. Horm Res 2008;70(1):51–7.
88. Monteleone P, Maj M. Dysfunctions of leptin, ghrelin, BDNF and endocannabinoids in eating disorders: beyond the homeostatic control of food intake. Psychoneuroendocrinology 2013;38(3):312–30.
89. Legroux-Gerot I, Vignau J, Biver E, et al. Anorexia nervosa, osteoporosis and circulating leptin: the missing link. Osteoporos Int 2010;21(10):1715–22.
90. Muller TD, Focker M, Holtkamp K, et al. Leptin-mediated neuroendocrine alterations in anorexia nervosa: somatic and behavioral implications. Child Adolesc Psychiatr Clin N Am 2009;18(1):117–29.
91. Monteleone P, DiLieto A, Castaldo E, et al. Leptin functioning in eating disorders. CNS Spectr 2004;9(7):523–9.
92. Mitan LA. Menstrual dysfunction in anorexia nervosa. J Pediatr Adolesc Gynecol 2004;17(2):81–5.
93. Chou SH, Mantzoros C. Bone metabolism in anorexia nervosa and hypothalamic amenorrhea. Metabolism 2018;80:91–104.
94. Chou SH, Chamberland JP, Liu X, et al. Leptin is an effective treatment for hypothalamic amenorrhea. Proc Natl Acad Sci U S A 2011;108(16):6585–90.
95. Welt CK, Chan JL, Bullen J, et al. Recombinant human leptin in women with hypothalamic amenorrhea. N Engl J Med 2004;351(10):987–97.
96. Chan JL, Mantzoros CS. Role of leptin in energy-deprivation states: normal human physiology and clinical implications for hypothalamic amenorrhoea and anorexia nervosa. Lancet 2005;366(9479):74–85.
97. Kosmiski L, Schmiege SJ, Mascolo M, et al. Chronic starvation secondary to anorexia nervosa is associated with an adaptive suppression of resting energy expenditure. J Clin Endocrinol Metab 2014;99(3):908–14.
98. Krahn DD, Rock C, Dechert RE, et al. Changes in resting energy expenditure and body composition in anorexia nervosa patients during refeeding. J Am Diet Assoc 1993;93(4):434–8.
99. Vaisman N, Rossi MF, Goldberg E, et al. Energy expenditure and body composition in patients with anorexia nervosa. J Pediatr 1988;113(5):919–24.
100. Kaye WH, Gwirtsman HE, Obarzanek E, et al. Caloric intake necessary for weight maintenance in anorexia nervosa: nonbulimics require greater caloric intake than bulimics. Am J Clin Nutr 1986;44(4):435–43.
101. Dempsey DT, Crosby LO, Pertschuk MJ, et al. Weight gain and nutritional efficacy in anorexia nervosa. Am J Clin Nutr 1984;39(2):236–42.
102. Gwirtsman HE, Kaye WH, Obarzanek E, et al. Decreased caloric intake in normal-weight patients with bulimia: comparison with female volunteers. Am J Clin Nutr 1989;49(1):86–92.

103. Konrad KK, Carels RA, Garner DM. Metabolic and psychological changes during refeeding in anorexia nervosa. Eat Weight Disord 2007;12(1):20–6.
104. Forman-Hoffman VL, Ruffin T, Schultz SK. Basal metabolic rate in anorexia nervosa patients: using appropriate predictive equations during the refeeding process. Ann Clin Psychiatry 2006;18(2):123–7.
105. Obarzanek E, Lesem MD, Jimerson DC. Resting metabolic rate of anorexia nervosa patients during weight gain. Am J Clin Nutr 1994;60(5):666–75.
106. Peebles R, Lesser A, Park CC, et al. Outcomes of an inpatient medical nutritional rehabilitation protocol in children and adolescents with eating disorders. J Eat Disord 2017;5:7.
107. Cleary BS, Gaudiani JL, Mehler PS. Interpreting the complete blood count in anorexia nervosa. Eat Disord 2010;18(2):132–9.
108. De Filippo E, Marra M, Alfinito F, et al. Hematological complications in anorexia nervosa. Eur J Clin Nutr 2016;70(11):1305–8.
109. Ecklund K, Vajapeyam S, Mulkern RV, et al. Bone marrow fat content in 70 adolescent girls with anorexia nervosa: magnetic resonance imaging and magnetic resonance spectroscopy assessment. Pediatr Radiol 2017;47(8):952–62.
110. Hutter G, Ganepola S, Hofmann WK. The hematology of anorexia nervosa. Int J Eat Disord 2009;42(4):293–300.
111. Pham-Scottez A. Medical complications of anorexia nervosa. Rev Prat 2016; 66(2):153–7 [in French].
112. Schafernak KT. Gelatinous transformation of the bone marrow from anorexia nervosa. Blood 2016;127(10):1374.
113. Devuyst O, Lambert M, Rodhain J, et al. Haematological changes and infectious complications in anorexia nervosa: a case-control study. Q J Med 1993;86(12): 791–9.
114. Marcos A, Varela P, Santacruz I, et al. Nutritional status and immunocompetence in eating disorders. A comparative study. Eur J Clin Nutr 1993;47(11):787–93.
115. Hariz A, Hamdi MS, Boukhris I, et al. Gelatinous transformation of bone marrow in a patient with anorexia nervosa: an uncommon but reversible etiology. Am J Case Rep 2018;19:1449–52.
116. Takeshima M, Ishikawa H, Kitadate A, et al. Anorexia nervosa-associated pancytopenia mimicking idiopathic aplastic anemia: a case report. BMC Psychiatry 2018;18(1):150.
117. Anyan WR Jr. Changes in erythrocyte sedimentation rate and fibrinogen during anorexia nervosa. J Pediatr 1974;85(4):525–7.
118. Pincherle G, Shanks J. Value of the erythrocyte sedimentation rate as a screening test. Br J Prev Soc Med 1967;21(3):133–6.
119. Amianto F, Caroppo P, D'Agata F, et al. Brain volumetric abnormalities in patients with anorexia and bulimia nervosa: a voxel-based morphometry study. Psychiatry Res 2013;213(3):210–6.
120. Fonville L, Giampietro V, Williams SC, et al. Alterations in brain structure in adults with anorexia nervosa and the impact of illness duration. Psychol Med 2014; 44(9):1965–75.
121. Fujisawa TX, Yatsuga C, Mabe H, et al. Anorexia nervosa during adolescence is associated with decreased gray matter volume in the inferior frontal gyrus. PLoS One 2015;10(6):e0128548.
122. King JA, Geisler D, Ritschel F, et al. Global cortical thinning in acute anorexia nervosa normalizes following long-term weight restoration. Biol Psychiatry 2015;77(7):624–32.

123. Martin Monzon B, Henderson LA, Madden S, et al. Grey matter volume in adolescents with anorexia nervosa and associated eating disorder symptoms. Eur J Neurosci 2017;46(7):2297–307.
124. Seitz J, Buhren K, von Polier GG, et al. Morphological changes in the brain of acutely ill and weight-recovered patients with anorexia nervosa. A meta-analysis and qualitative review. Z Kinder Jugendpsychiatr Psychother 2014; 42(1):7–17 [quiz 17–8].
125. Seitz J, Walter M, Mainz V, et al. Brain volume reduction predicts weight development in adolescent patients with anorexia nervosa. J Psychiatr Res 2015;68: 228–37.
126. Allen KL, Byrne SM, Hii H, et al. Neurocognitive functioning in adolescents with eating disorders: a population-based study. Cogn Neuropsychiatry 2013;18(5): 355–75.
127. Brand M, Franke-Sievert C, Jacoby GE, et al. Neuropsychological correlates of decision making in patients with bulimia nervosa. Neuropsychology 2007;21(6): 742–50.
128. Buhren K, Mainz V, Herpertz-Dahlmann B, et al. Cognitive flexibility in juvenile anorexia nervosa patients before and after weight recovery. J Neural Transm (Vienna) 2012;119(9):1047–57.
129. Darcy AM, Fitzpatrick KK, Colborn D, et al. Set-shifting among adolescents with bulimic spectrum eating disorders. Psychosom Med 2012;74(8):869–72.
130. Fowler L, Blackwell A, Jaffa A, et al. Profile of neurocognitive impairments associated with female in-patients with anorexia nervosa. Psychol Med 2006;36(4): 517–27.
131. Galderisi S, Bucci P, Mucci A, et al. Neurocognitive functioning in bulimia nervosa: the role of neuroendocrine, personality and clinical aspects. Psychol Med 2011;41(4):839–48.
132. Galimberti E, Fadda E, Cavallini MC, et al. Executive functioning in anorexia nervosa patients and their unaffected relatives. Psychiatry Res 2013;208(3): 238–44.
133. Guillaume S, Gorwood P, Jollant F, et al. Impaired decision-making in symptomatic anorexia and bulimia nervosa patients: a meta-analysis. Psychol Med 2015; 45(16):3377–91.
134. Kjaersdam Telleus G, Jepsen JR, Bentz M, et al. Cognitive profile of children and adolescents with anorexia nervosa. Eur Eat Disord Rev 2015;23(1):34–42.
135. Lang K, Stahl D, Espie J, et al. Set shifting in children and adolescents with anorexia nervosa: an exploratory systematic review and meta-analysis. Int J Eat Disord 2014;47(4):394–9.
136. McAnarney ER, Zarcone J, Singh P, et al. Restrictive anorexia nervosa and set-shifting in adolescents: a biobehavioral interface. J Adolesc Health 2011;49(1): 99–101.
137. Roberts ME, Tchanturia K, Treasure JL. Exploring the neurocognitive signature of poor set-shifting in anorexia and bulimia nervosa. J Psychiatr Res 2010; 44(14):964–70.
138. Brown M, Loeb KL, McGrath RE, et al. Executive functioning and central coherence in anorexia nervosa: pilot investigation of a neurocognitive endophenotype. Eur Eat Disord Rev 2018;26(5):489–98.
139. Penas-Lledo EM, Loeb KL, Martin L, et al. Anterior cingulate activity in bulimia nervosa: a fMRI case study. Eat Weight Disord 2007;12(4):e78–82.
140. Weinbach N, Sher H, Lock JD, et al. Attention networks in adolescent anorexia nervosa. Eur Child Adolesc Psychiatry 2018;27(3):343–51.

141. Chui HT, Christensen BK, Zipursky RB, et al. Cognitive function and brain structure in females with a history of adolescent-onset anorexia nervosa. Pediatrics 2008;122(2):e426–37.
142. Gainotti G. Anosognosia, denial of illness and the right hemisphere dominance for emotions: some historical and clinical notes. Conscious Cogn 2018;58: 44–50.
143. Lask B, Frampton I. Anorexia nervosa–irony, misnomer and paradox. Eur Eat Disord Rev 2009;17(3):165–8.
144. Denholm M, Jankowski J. Gastroesophageal reflux disease and bulimia nervosa–a review of the literature. Dis Esophagus 2011;24(2):79–85.
145. Garcia Garcia B, Dean Ferrer A, Diaz Jimenez N, et al. Bilateral parotid Sialadenosis associated with long-standing bulimia: a case report and literature review. J Maxillofac Oral Surg 2018;17(2):117–21.
146. Hochlehnert A, Lowe B, Bludau HB, et al. Spontaneous pneumomediastinum in anorexia nervosa: a case report and review of the literature on pneumomediastinum and pneumothorax. Eur Eat Disord Rev 2010;18(2):107–15.
147. Jensen VM, Stoving RK, Andersen PE. Anorexia nervosa with massive pulmonary air leak and extraordinary propagation. Int J Eat Disord 2017;50(4):451–3.
148. McCurdy JM, McKenzie CE, El-Mallakh RS. Recurrent subcutaneous emphysema as a consequence of bulimia nervosa. Int J Eat Disord 2013;46(1):92–4.
149. Paszynska E, Slopien A, Weglarz M, et al. Parotid salivary parameters in bulimic patients - a controlled clinical trial. Psychiatr Pol 2015;49(4):709–20.
150. Romanos GE, Javed F, Romanos EB, et al. Oro-facial manifestations in patients with eating disorders. Appetite 2012;59(2):499–504.
151. Weterle-Smolinska KA, Banasiuk M, Dziekiewicz M, et al. Gastrointestinal motility disorders in patients with anorexia nervosa - a review of the literature. Psychiatria polska 2015;49(4):721–9.
152. Fong HF, Divasta AD, Difabio D, et al. Prevalence and predictors of abnormal liver enzymes in young women with anorexia nervosa. J Pediatr 2008;153(2): 247–53.
153. Gwee K, Teh A, Huang C. Acute superior mesenteric artery syndrome and pancreatitis in anorexia nervosa. Australas Psychiatry 2010;18(6):523–6.
154. Nagata JM, Park KT, Colditz K, et al. Associations of elevated liver enzymes among hospitalized adolescents with anorexia nervosa. J Pediatr 2015;166(2): 439–43.e1.
155. Rosen E, Bakshi N, Watters A, et al. Hepatic complications of anorexia nervosa. Dig Dis Sci 2017;62(11):2977–81.
156. Urso C, Brucculeri S, Caimi G. Marked elevation of transaminases and pancreatic enzymes in severe malnourished male with eating disorder. Clin Ter 2013; 164(5):e387–91.
157. Weinbrenner T, Zuger M, Jacoby GE, et al. Lipoprotein metabolism in patients with anorexia nervosa: a case-control study investigating the mechanisms leading to hypercholesterolaemia. Br J Nutr 2004;91(6):959–69.
158. Matzkin VB, Geissler C, Coniglio R, et al. Cholesterol concentrations in patients with Anorexia Nervosa and in healthy controls. Int J Psychiatr Nurs Res 2006; 11(2):1283–93.
159. Monteleone P, Santonastaso P, Pannuto M, et al. Enhanced serum cholesterol and triglyceride levels in bulimia nervosa: relationships to psychiatric comorbidity, psychopathology and hormonal variables. Psychiatry Res 2005;134(3): 267–73.

160. Moschonis G, Georgiou A, Sarapi K, et al. Association of distorted eating behaviors with cardiometabolic risk indices in preadolescents. The Healthy Growth Study. Appetite 2015;91:35–40.

161. Nakai Y, Noma S, Fukusima M, et al. Serum lipid levels in patients with eating disorders. Intern Med 2016;55(14):1853–7.

162. Elbadaway MH. Chronic superior mesenteric artery syndrome in anorexia nervosa. Br J Psychiatry 1992;160:552–4.

163. Antic M, Ghodduci KM, Brussaard C, et al. Massive gastric dilatation in bulimic patient. JBR-BTR 2014;97(3):136–7.

164. Birmingham CL, Boone S. Pancreatitis causing death in bulimia nervosa. Int J Eat Disord 2004;36(2):234–7.

165. Bravender T, Story L. Massive binge eating, gastric dilatation and unsuccessful purging in a young woman with bulimia nervosa. J Adolesc Health 2007;41(5): 516–8.

166. Dewangan M, Khare MK, Mishra S, et al. Binge eating leading to acute gastric dilatation, ischemic necrosis and rupture -a case report. J Clin Diagn Res 2016; 10(3):Pd06–7.

167. Dincel O, Goksu M. Acute gastric dilatation due to binge eating may be fatal. North Clin Istanb 2017;4(2):199–202.

168. Garcia Vasquez C, Cortes Guiral D, Rivas Fidalgo S, et al. Gigantic gastric retention due to bulimic binge eating. Cir Esp 2014;92(6):e33.

169. Kim HH, Park SJ, Park MI, et al. Acute gastric dilatation and acute pancreatitis in a patient with an eating disorder: solving a chicken and egg situation. Intern Med 2011;50(6):571–5.

170. Marano AR, Sangree MH. Acute pancreatitis associated with bulimia. J Clin Gastroenterol 1984;6(3):245–8.

171. Maung H, Buxey KN, Studd C, et al. Acute gastric dilatation in a bulimic patient. Gastrointest Endosc 2017;85(2):455–7.

172. Morris LG, Stephenson KE, Herring S, et al. Recurrent acute pancreatitis in anorexia and bulimia. JOP 2004;5(4):231–4.

173. Nam K, Shin HD, Shin JE. Acute gastric dilatation and ischemia associated with portal vein gas caused by binge eating. Korean J Intern Med 2019;34(1):231–2.

174. Panach-Navarrete J, Moro-Valdezate D, Garces-Albir M, et al. Acute gastric dilatation in the context of bulimia nervosa. Rev Esp Enferm Dig 2015;107(9): 580–1.

175. Evrard F, da Cunha MP, Lambert M, et al. Impaired osmoregulation in anorexia nervosa: a case-control study. Nephrol Dial Transplant 2004;19(12):3034–9.

176. Kanbur N, Katzman DK. Impaired osmoregulation in anorexia nervosa: review of the literature. Pediatr Endocrinol Rev 2011;8(3):218–21.

177. Stheneur C, Bergeron S, Lapeyraque AL. Renal complications in anorexia nervosa. Eat Weight Disord 2014;19(4):455–60.

178. Stheneur C, Bergeron SJ, Frappier JY, et al. Renal injury in pediatric anorexia nervosa: a retrospective study. Eat Weight Disord 2019;24(2):323–7.

179. Cariem AK, Lemmer ER, Adams MG, et al. Severe hypophosphataemia in anorexia nervosa. Postgrad Med J 1994;70(829):825–7.

180. Greenfeld D, Mickley D, Quinlan DM, et al. Hypokalemia in outpatients with eating disorders. Am J Psychiatry 1995;152(1):60–3.

181. Khardori R. Refeeding syndrome and hypophosphatemia. J Intensive Care Med 2005;20(3):174–5.

182. Peeters F, Meijboom A. Electrolyte and other blood serum abnormalities in normal weight bulimia nervosa: evidence for sampling bias. Int J Eat Disord 2000;27(3):358–62.

183. Wolfe BE, Metzger ED, Levine JM, et al. Laboratory screening for electrolyte abnormalities and anemia in bulimia nervosa: a controlled study. Int J Eat Disord 2001;30(3):288–93.

184. Mehler PS, Blalock DV, Walden K, et al. Medical findings in 1,026 consecutive adult inpatient-residential eating disordered patients. Int J Eat Disord 2018; 51(4):305–13.

185. Marinella MA. Refeeding syndrome and hypophosphatemia. J Intensive Care Med 2005;20(3):155–9.

186. O'Connor G, Nicholls D. Refeeding hypophosphatemia in adolescents with anorexia nervosa: a systematic review. Nutr Clin Pract 2013;28(3):358–64.

187. Ornstein RM, Golden NH, Jacobson MS, et al. Hypophosphatemia during nutritional rehabilitation in anorexia nervosa: implications for refeeding and monitoring. J Adolesc Health 2003;32(1):83–8.

188. Skipper A. Refeeding syndrome or refeeding hypophosphatemia: a systematic review of cases. Nutr Clin Pract 2012;27(1):34–40.

189. Hall RC, Hoffman RS, Beresford TP, et al. Hypomagnesemia in patients with eating disorders. Psychosomatics 1988;29(3):264–72.

190. Norris ML, Pinhas L, Nadeau PO, et al. Delirium and refeeding syndrome in anorexia nervosa. Int J Eat Disord 2012;45(3):439–42.

191. O'Connor G, Goldin J. The refeeding syndrome and glucose load. Int J Eat Disord 2011;44(2):182–5.

192. Ormerod C, Farrer K, Harper L, et al. Refeeding syndrome: a clinical review. Br J Hosp Med (Lond) 2010;71(12):686–90.

193. Solomon SM, Kirby DF. The refeeding syndrome: a review. JPEN J Parenter Enteral Nutr 1990;14(1):90–7.

194. Viana Lde A, Burgos MG, Silva Rde A. Refeeding syndrome: clinical and nutritional relevance. Arq Bras Cir Dig 2012;25(1):56–9.

195. Walmsley RS. Refeeding syndrome: screening, incidence, and treatment during parenteral nutrition. J Gastroenterol Hepatol 2013;28(Suppl 4):113–7.

196. Mehanna HM, Moledina J, Travis J. Refeeding syndrome: what it is, and how to prevent and treat it. BMJ 2008;336(7659):1495–8.

197. Setnick J. Micronutrient deficiencies and supplementation in anorexia and bulimia nervosa: a review of literature. Nutr Clin Pract 2010;25(2):137–42.

198. Fisher M, Simpser E, Schneider M. Hypophosphatemia secondary to oral refeeding in anorexia nervosa. Int J Eat Disord 2000;28(2):181–7.

199. Santonastaso P, Sala A, Favaro A. Water intoxication in anorexia nervosa: a case report. Int J Eat Disord 1998;24(4):439–42.

200. Cuesta MJ, Juan JA, Peralta V. Secondary seizures from water intoxication in anorexia nervosa. Gen Hosp Psychiatry 1992;14(3):212–3.

201. Miller KK, Grinspoon SK, Ciampa J, et al. Medical findings in outpatients with anorexia nervosa. Arch Intern Med 2005;165(5):561–6.

202. Ramli M, Hassan AS, Rosnani S. Dissociative episode secondary to hypoglycemic state in anorexia nervosa: a case report. Int J Eat Disord 2009;42(3):290–2.

203. Yamada Y, Fushimi H, Inoue T, et al. Anorexia nervosa with recurrent hypoglycemic coma and cerebral hemorrhage. Intern Med 1996;35(7):560–3.

204. Yanai H, Yoshida H, Tomono Y, et al. Severe hypoglycemia in a patient with anorexia nervosa. Eat Weight Disord 2008;13(1):e1–3.

205. Yasuhara D, Deguchi D, Tsutsui J, et al. A characteristic reactive hypoglycemia induced by rapid change of eating behavior in anorexia nervosa: a case report. Int J Eat Disord 2003;34(2):273–7.
206. Yasuhara D, Kojima S, Nozoe S, et al. Intense fear of caloric intake related to severe hypoglycemia in anorexia nervosa. Gen Hosp Psychiatry 2004;26(3): 243–5.
207. Barron LJ, Barron RF, Johnson JCS, et al. A retrospective analysis of biochemical and haematological parameters in patients with eating disorders. J Eat Disord 2017;5:32.
208. Gatti D, El Ghoch M, Viapiana O, et al. Strong relationship between vitamin D status and bone mineral density in anorexia nervosa. Bone 2015;78:212–5.
209. Hanachi M, Dicembre M, Rives-Lange C, et al. Micronutrients deficiencies in 374 severely malnourished anorexia nervosa inpatients. Nutrients 2019;11(4) [pii:E792].
210. Modan-Moses D, Levy-Shraga Y, Pinhas-Hamiel O, et al. High prevalence of vitamin D deficiency and insufficiency in adolescent inpatients diagnosed with eating disorders. Int J Eat Disord 2015;48(6):607–14.
211. Renthal W, Marin-Valencia I, Evans PA. Thiamine deficiency secondary to anorexia nervosa: an uncommon cause of peripheral neuropathy and Wernicke encephalopathy in adolescence. Pediatr Neurol 2014;51(1):100–3.
212. Golden NH, Katzman DK, Sawyer SM, et al. Position Paper of the Society for Adolescent Health and Medicine: medical management of restrictive eating disorders in adolescents and young adults. J Adolesc Health 2015;56(1):121–5.
213. Becker P, Carney LN, Corkins MR, et al. Consensus statement of the Academy of Nutrition and Dietetics/American Society for Parenteral and Enteral Nutrition: indicators recommended for the identification and documentation of pediatric malnutrition (undernutrition). Nutr Clin Pract 2015;30(1):147–61.
214. Garber AK, Mauldin K, Michihata N, et al. Higher calorie diets increase rate of weight gain and shorten hospital stay in hospitalized adolescents with anorexia nervosa. J Adolesc Health 2013;53(5):579–84.
215. Garber AK, Michihata N, Hetnal K, et al. A prospective examination of weight gain in hospitalized adolescents with anorexia nervosa on a recommended refeeding protocol. J Adolesc Health 2012;50(1):24–9.
216. Garber AK, Sawyer SM, Golden NH, et al. A systematic review of approaches to refeeding in patients with anorexia nervosa. Int J Eat Disord 2016;49(3): 293–310.
217. Madden S, Miskovic-Wheatley J, Clarke S, et al. Outcomes of a rapid refeeding protocol in adolescent anorexia nervosa. J Eat Disord 2015;3:8.
218. R. Peebles, L. Collins Lyster-Mensh and R.E. Kreipe. Eating disorders. In: K. R. Ginsburg, S. B. Kinsman, eds. Reaching teens: strength-based communication strategies to build resilience and support healthy adolescent development (a textbook and video product). American Academy of Pediatrics, Elks Grove Village, IL, January 2014.
219. Gentile MG, Lessa C, Cattaneo M. Metabolic and nutritional needs to normalize body mass index by doubling the admission body weight in severe anorexia nervosa. Clin Med Insights Case Rep 2013;6:51–6.

The Role of Puberty and Ovarian Hormones in the Genetic Diathesis of Eating Disorders in Females

Ruofan Ma, BMath[a,1], Megan E. Mikhail, BS[a],
Natasha Fowler, MA[a], Kristen M. Culbert, PhD[b],
Kelly L. Klump, PhD[c],*

KEYWORDS

- Puberty • Eating disorders • Anorexia nervosa • Bulimia nervosa
- Binge eating disorder • Binge eating • Progesterone • Estrogen

KEY POINTS

- Incidence of eating disorders increases and becomes female predominant after puberty. Although traditional etiologic models have often focused on the influence of psychosocial risk factors, accumulating evidence indicates a role for biological/genetic influence in these increases.
- Genetic influences on disordered eating increase dramatically during puberty in girls.
- Increases in ovarian hormones, particularly estrogen, may account for these increases in genetic effects.
- Properly communicating the role of genetics and other biological factors in the cause of eating disorders has the potential to reduce stigma for individuals suffering from these conditions.

INTRODUCTION

Puberty is a critical risk period for the development of eating disorders in girls.[1] Although disturbances in behaviors related to eating and weight have been documented in pre-adolescent females,[2] most full-syndromal eating disorders (ie, anorexia

Conflicts of Interest: The authors have no conflicts of interest to disclose.
[a] Department of Psychology, Michigan State University, 316 Physics Road, Room 43, East Lansing, MI 48824, USA; [b] Department of Psychology, University of Nevada, Las Vegas, 4505 Maryland Parkway, Las Vegas, NV 89154-5030, USA; [c] Department of Psychology, Michigan State University, 316 Physics Road, Room 107B, East Lansing, MI 48824-1116, USA
[1] Present address: 20 Bruyeres Mews, Unit 2007, Toronto, Ontario M5V 0G8, Canada.
* Corresponding author.
E-mail address: klump@msu.edu

nervosa [AN], bulimia nervosa [BN], binge eating disorder [BED] and other specified feeding and eating disorders [OSFEDs]) rarely onset before puberty.[3] Symptoms of disordered eating (ie, body dissatisfaction, weight/shape concerns, dietary restraint, dieting, binge eating, purging behaviors) become much more prevalent during puberty and in post-puberty than in pre-puberty in girls.[1] Although no sex differences in disordered eating are observed before puberty, the female to male ratio for disordered eating symptoms ranges from 2:1 to 10:1 after puberty.[3]

Traditional theories have posited psychosocial factors as major contributors to these sex differences and pubertal increases in risk for disordered eating in girls.[4] For instance, physical changes in girls during puberty create discrepancies between their body shape and the "thin ideal," whereas physical changes in boys may be seen as a progression toward an ideal body shape associated with more masculinity.[4] This difference in beauty ideals between the sexes has been posited to cause increased body dissatisfaction and negative mood and decreased self-esteem in girls, all of which elevate risk for eating-related disturbances.[4] However, this conceptualization has undergone considerable transformations in the last decades with increasing recognition of biological influences in the cause of disordered eating. Current theories have reached a tentative consensus that a comprehensive risk model of eating disorders and their symptoms should represent a true integration of biological and psychosocial factors.[5]

Genetic factors and ovarian hormones are emerging as two key biological factors that contribute to pubertal risk.[6,7] Indeed, the past several years have been marked by a notable increase in the number of studies examining the intersection of genetic and hormonal factors in the development of disordered eating. The aim of this review is to summarize these data and suggest directions for future research. We begin with descriptions of phenotypic associations between puberty and disordered eating and sex differences in these associations. We then review data suggesting that genetic and hormonal factors may contribute to sex-differentiated eating behaviors during and after puberty. Where appropriate, we review results from both human and animal studies in order to capitalize on the ecological validity of human studies and the strong experimental rigor that is present in animal work. Finally, we discuss clinical implications and summarize future research directions for disentangling genetic and hormonal mechanisms in pubertal risk for disordered eating.

PHENOTYPIC ASSOCIATIONS BETWEEN PUBERTY AND DISORDERED EATING

Cross-sectional, longitudinal/prospective, and/or retrospective studies have differentiated pubertal status (ie, pubertal stage at a given point in time, such as pre-puberty vs post-puberty) from pubertal timing (ie, onset of puberty relative to peers, such as early, on-time, vs late maturation) effects when examining risk periods for eating disorders. Data from both perspectives consistently implicate puberty as a critical risk period for eating disorders in girls, particularly in regard to BN, BED, and OSFEDs.[1,3,6] In terms of pubertal status, girls at more advanced stages of pubertal development have significantly increased rates of these disorders, even after controlling for age.[3] In terms of pubertal timing, compared with women without eating disorders, a higher percentage of women with these disorders also experienced early pubertal maturation.[3] Although there is less consistent support for pubertal risk for development of AN, onset of AN is nevertheless rare before puberty.[3] The less consistent evidence for pubertal risk for AN may be due to its associated extreme dieting, which usually begins months before full criteria for AN are met and may forestall pubertal development.[8,9] This complex entanglement between extreme dieting and developmental growth makes it challenging to determine the directionality of effects between AN and puberty.

However, there is significant overlap in symptomology between different eating disorder diagnoses, so using global measures of disordered eating symptoms (eg, body dissatisfaction, weight/shape concerns, binge eating, dietary restraint, and purging behaviors) may yield transdiagnostic insights that contribute to understanding AN despite its low prevalence and physiologic complexity. Although binge eating is frequently associated with BN and BED, it is also a characteristic of the AN binge eating/purging subtype.[3] Strict dieting, commonly associated with AN, is characteristic of BN as well.[3] Several other symptoms, such as exaggerated concern with weight gain, dietary restraint, body dissatisfaction, and body image distortion, are present in all types of eating disorders.[10] In fact, approximately 50% of women with AN develop BN during the course of their illness, and about 30% of women with BN have met criteria for AN at some point.[11–13] With significant overlap in symptoms and accumulating evidence that eating disorders may be more appropriately classified with dimensional rather than categorical approaches,[14] studies have increasingly used global measures of disordered eating symptoms. Disordered eating symptoms also are more prevalent than eating disorders, and thus, using these global measures allows for larger sample sizes and greater statistical power to detect effects while helping to identify early indicators of the potential development of full-blown eating disorders.

Numerous studies using these symptom measures have shown that disordered eating is strongly associated with pubertal development in girls.[1] Rates of disordered eating symptoms tend to be higher among girls at more advanced pubertal stages or who exhibit earlier pubertal maturation, compared with girls at earlier pubertal stages or who mature later. For example, in a study that compared eating-related behaviors and attitudes in 11-year-old girls by stages of pubertal maturation, post-menarcheal girls endorsed significantly more dieting and increased body image dissatisfaction than pre-menarcheal girls.[15] It remains unknown, however, whether pubertal status (ie, pre-puberty, puberty, post-puberty) and pubertal timing (ie, early, on-time, late maturation) both independently affect disordered eating or whether one contributes more critically than the other. Despite this uncertainty, the current literature overall presents strong support for the significance of pubertal processes in disordered eating in girls.[1]

Interestingly, these same pubertal effects have been observed in female rats. Animal models can further disentangle genetic from environmental and psychosocial influences on eating behaviors because animals do not experience key psychosocial risk factors (eg, body image concerns) that may affect humans. To date, only two studies[16,17] have used animal models to examine the effects of puberty on risk for disordered eating symptoms. One study followed samples of female rats longitudinally from pre-puberty to adulthood and examined whether binge eating proneness (ie, the tendency to consistently consume larger amounts of food high in fat and/or sugar in a short period of time) would emerge during puberty. Rats were identified as binge eating prone or resistant in adulthood, and then their rates of binge eating during pre-puberty and puberty were examined. No significant group differences in binge eating behaviors were observed in pre-puberty (ie, both binge eating prone and binge eating resistant rats consumed the same amount of palatable food during feeding tests). Starting in mid-late puberty, however, rates of binge eating increased significantly in the binge eating prone rats as compared with the binge eating resistant rats. These results were replicated across two independent samples of rats in this study and have now been replicated in another study.[17] These findings further highlight the role of biological factors in individual differences in disordered eating symptoms across pubertal development, independent of traditionally emphasized psychosocial factors.

Although there is strong support in the literature for pubertal effects on disordered eating in females, relatively few studies have been conducted in males, and results thus far seem to be less consistent than those in females. Specifically, although some studies have found positive associations between pubertal status/timing and body dissatisfaction in males,[1] a substantial number of studies have reported no such effects.[1,18–20] A meta-analysis that examined associations between pubertal timing and disordered eating showed significant pubertal timing effects in girls but only small and marginally significant effects in boys.[21] Only one animal study has examined pubertal influences on binge eating proneness in male rats. Average rates of binge eating proneness were similar in pre-pubertal and pubertal male rats, whereas rates of binge eating proneness increased in female rats after pubertal onset.[17] Given that most studies have focused on the role of puberty in disordered eating in girls, in the following discussion we focus on mechanisms underlying pubertal processes in girls and only include data from studies in males when appropriate.

GENETIC AND HORMONAL FACTORS

The robust associations between puberty and eating disorders as well as disordered eating symptoms in girls have led to efforts to identify factors underlying these phenotypic changes during puberty. Emerging data from twin studies suggest that genetic and hormonal factors may be critical mechanisms.[7,22–24]

Genetic Factors

Initial hints that genetic factors might be important for pubertal risk for disordered eating came from developmental twin studies showing age differences in genetic effects.[25,26] Although genetic influence is often thought to be fixed across the lifespan, studies from various fields of psychology (eg, cognitive psychology) have shown that the degree of genetic influence on a disorder or trait varies across time.[27] For example, for individuals not growing up in disadvantaged contexts,[28,29] genetic effects account for little variance in intelligence quotient (IQ) scores during childhood, but as individuals mature, genes become increasingly important and account for more than 50% of the variance in IQ in adulthood.[27] These changes may be due to biological maturation, changes in environment, or the accumulating effects of bidirectional gene-environment influences.[27] Similarly, the extent to which disordered eating is influenced by genetic factors may differ across development, especially given the increase in prevalence of eating disorders during adolescence in girls described earlier.

Using both cross-sectional[26,30] and longitudinal[25,31,32] designs, twin studies have demonstrated significant increases in genetic influences on disordered eating across adolescence in females. These increases have been observed when using measures of both overall disordered eating and individual symptoms (eg, weight and shape concerns). For example, in a longitudinal twin study across ages 11, 14, and 18 years, negligible genetic influences (6% heritability) were observed on a global measure of disordered eating symptoms (ie, assessing body dissatisfaction, weight preoccupation, binge eating, and use of compensatory behaviors) at age 11 years.[25] However, between ages 11 and 14 years, genetic effects on disordered eating increased to greater than or equal to 45%, and this percentage remained constant from ages 14 to 18 years. A second longitudinal study assessed adolescent twins during three age periods (12–13, 13–15, 14–16 years) and found increasing genetic influence on weight and shape concerns between ages 12 and 15 years but not in later adolescence.[32] Finally, in a cross-sectional study that combined data from three twin registries in the United States and Australia,[26] the heritability of weight and shape concerns again increased dramatically from age 11 (0%) to age 14 years (54%), but then remained constant from age 14 years into middle adulthood (ie, age 41 years). There are some data suggesting that there are no new genetic factors that come on-line after mid-adolescence in female twins,[25] although other data suggest that there may be new sources of genetic variation in later adolescence.[31] Clearly, these later inconsistent results require additional study, but overall, there is strong support for the presence of significant increases in genetic effects on disordered eating across adolescent ages that mirror developmental patterns of symptom emergence. Early-to-mid adolescence in girls seems to be a particularly important risk period, during which rates of disordered eating increase and genetic factors become much more prominent.

Differences across puberty

The average age of menarche in the United States (ie, age 12.5 years)[33] overlaps with the developmental period (ie, ages 11–14 years)[25] during which genetic effects on disordered eating significantly increase in girls. Thus, rather than age per se, pubertal development, which is associated with biological changes conceivably contributing to genetic effects, may be the critical factor underlying the increase in heritability of disordered eating observed during early adolescence.[34] Several cross-sectional twin studies have now confirmed that puberty, rather than age, contributes to increases in genetic effects across adolescence. These studies have shown dramatic increases in genetic effects across puberty in girls, with 0% heritability of a range of disordered eating symptoms (ie, global measures, as well as measures of binge eating, shape/weight concerns, etc.)[34–37] in pre-early puberty and ~50% heritability in mid-to-late puberty and beyond.[34–37] All studies controlled for the effects of age (for example, by examining girls who were at the same age but differed in pubertal development).[34–37] Findings generally suggest that mid-puberty is a particularly key time for the increase in genetic effects,[34–36] although there are studies suggesting linear increases in genetic effects across the full pubertal period.[35–37] Importantly, it is now recognized that shifts in genetic effects are not observed when using only very late indicators of pubertal development (ie, menarche only),[38] as differences in genetic effects occur earlier in the pubertal process (ie, between pre-early and mid-puberty).[35] Finally, studies of pubertal timing (ie, early vs late maturation, relative to peers)[39,40] further corroborate the importance of puberty in associations between genetic influence and disordered eating. Two twin studies have shown that a shared set of genetic factors accounts for phenotypic associations between early pubertal timing and disordered eating symptoms (ie, drive for thinness, a combined measure of binge eating/vomiting, body dissatisfaction, and dieting).[39,40] That is, genetic factors that contribute to girls' pubertal timing also contribute to disordered eating symptoms. Importantly, early puberty and the tendency to diet were no longer associated phenotypically when the shared genetic factors were statistically controlled,[40] suggesting that the association between pubertal timing and dieting is entirely due to genetic (rather than environmental) influences.[40] These findings add to those showing changes in genetic effects across puberty by confirming that genetic factors are the missing link in associations between pubertal development and disordered eating in girls.

Overall, the current literature provides strong support for puberty, rather than age per se, as a key developmental factor accounting for increases in genetic influences on disordered eating across adolescence in females. Furthermore, because eating disorder symptoms disproportionately affect females, the change mechanisms that expose adolescents to increased risk for disordered eating during puberty are likely to be sex specific. In fact, twin data have revealed stability in genetic influences on disordered eating (ie, a total score composed of body dissatisfaction, weight preoccupation, binge eating, and compensatory behaviors) in adolescent and adult male twins, where heritability has been estimated to be ~50% in puberty (ie, gonadarche) and young adulthood in males.[20] Instead, genetic effects on disordered eating in males seem to linearly increase during adrenarche, an early stage of puberty that occurs between ages 6 and 12 years and is marked by increasing androgens without any of the pubertal physical changes.[18] These potentially sex-differentiated processes of genetic effects during puberty may be driven by differences in hormone exposure across development, such as the activation of ovarian hormones in girls and androgen exposure in boys.[1,6,20,41] Although no studies have examined the role of androgens in genetic influence on disordered eating in boys, emerging evidence supports a role for ovarian hormones in pubertal differences in genetic effects in girls.

Ovarian Hormone Influences

Estrogen drives many biological changes associated with puberty in females, including the development of secondary sex characteristics (eg, breast development, hair growth, onset of menses).[42] Importantly, the developmental twin studies discussed earlier all relied on these secondary sex characteristics for assessing pubertal development.[34–36] Thus, changes in genetic risk for disordered eating across puberty may be the result of increasing estradiol levels. Although estradiol levels are low in pre-pubertal girls, they increase linearly across puberty,[42] closely mimicking the trajectory of increasing genetic effects on disordered eating during this period.[34–36] Progesterone (the other primary ovarian hormone) does not increase until after first ovulation, which occurs at a later stage of puberty than when the increases in genetic influence are observed. Thus, progesterone has been considered to be less likely to contribute to the changes in genetic effects observed during puberty,[1,41] and this impression has been confirmed in recent studies.[43] One primary function of estrogen is to regulate gene transcription in the central nervous system,[42,44] including neural pathways and systems that have been implicated in eating disorders (eg, serotonin, reward pathways involving dopamine and opioids).[45,46] Therefore, differential regulation of genetic expression in key neurobiological pathways may be an important pubertal mechanism through which estrogen drives increases in genetic influence on disordered eating.[42,44]

If estrogen plays a role in regulating transcription of genes related to disordered eating risk during puberty, then the extent to which genetic factors influence disordered eating would be expected to differ at varying levels of estradiol (ie, estradiol level should moderate genetic influences on disordered eating during puberty). Our research group has examined this possibility through two twin studies that compared the degree of genetic influence on disordered eating between individuals with higher versus lower estradiol levels during puberty. Both studies observed significant effects of estrogen on disordered eating symptoms in girls, although the results were in opposing directions. In a small-scale pilot study (N = 99 twin pairs; mean age = 11.98) of female twins,[41] stronger genetic influences were observed at higher versus lower estradiol levels for a range of disordered eating symptoms (ie, weight preoccupation, body dissatisfaction, a combined binge eating/compensatory behaviors scale, and the total score on the measure). By contrast, in a much larger follow-up study (N = 482 twin pairs; mean age = 11.75), genetic influences on binge eating symptoms were significantly stronger in girls with lower estradiol levels than in girls with higher estradiol levels.[7] In both studies, estradiol levels contributed to differences in genetic effects independent of age, body mass index, and secondary sex characteristics.

Discrepancies in study findings were puzzling but seemed to be related to differences in sample size and study methodology. The latter study used more sophisticated analytical techniques that enabled inclusion of all twin pairs in the analyses, including the pairs discordant on estradiol levels (ie, twin pairs in which one twin was high and the other was low in estrogen). The more powerful analyses and larger sample size may explain its differing results from the earlier pilot study. Importantly, findings in the larger study replicated across several within-study subsamples and ways of analyzing the data (ie, analyzing the pre-menarcheal twins only, analyzing the data with and without progesterone in the models, using single-day hormone values vs those across multiple days, etc.), suggesting that results were robust to sample composition, analytical methods, and study design decisions.[7]

Two recent adult twin studies[43,47] from our laboratory obtained findings that mirror results from the larger-scale investigation.[7] Using longitudinal twin data across the menstrual cycle, we found that genetic influences on emotional eating (ie, overeating in response to negative emotions, which is a precursor and strong correlate of binge eating) were 2 to 3 times higher in post-ovulation (ie, when estradiol levels are lower) than pre-ovulation (ie, when estradiol peaks).[47] Moreover, a cross-sectional study found significantly stronger genetic effects on emotional eating in women with lower estradiol levels as compared with women with higher estradiol levels.[43] Taken together, data from adolescence and adulthood provide relatively strong convergent evidence that lower levels of estradiol may be associated with increased genetic effects on binge eating and emotional eating across development. Mechanisms underlying these effects remain unknown, but estrogen is known to be protective against food intake and binge eating in adulthood in animals[48–51] and humans.[52–54] It may be that lower levels of estradiol during puberty disrupt normative pubertal processes and brain development and increase genetic effects and later phenotypic risk for binge eating in girls.[43] Clearly, additional animal and human studies are needed to examine these potential effects, but data thus far are converging in suggesting a prominent role for estrogen in genetic and phenotypic risk for disordered eating across development.[43]

FUTURE DIRECTIONS

Existing data provide strong support for puberty as a critical risk period for eating disorders and their symptoms in girls. Although sociocultural factors significantly contribute to development of disordered eating, accumulating data demonstrate the importance of genetic influence on these symptoms as well. As shown by developmental twin studies, genetic influences on disordered eating are dynamic and increase dramatically across adolescence, particularly during puberty. Ovarian hormones are prime candidates for explaining these developmental shifts, potentially through regulatory effects of estrogen on gene expression during puberty. Twin and animal studies suggest that secretions of estrogen during puberty may lead to differential trajectories of genetic effects on disordered eating and, potentially, the later development of full-blown eating disorders. More human and animal studies are clearly needed to replicate existing findings and confirm a role for estrogen in pubertal emergence of genetic influence and phenotypic presentations of disordered eating. Because most studies of estrogen effects have focused on binge eating or emotional eating only, more research is also needed to confirm whether the existing findings replicate across other disordered eating symptoms (eg, weight preoccupation, body dissatisfaction, and compensatory behaviors), particularly in humans in whom these symptoms can be examined/modeled much more easily than in animals.

Additional studies are also needed to identify specific neurobiological systems underlying pubertal and estrogen effects. Estrogen regulates gene transcription in many neurotransmitter/neurotrophin systems that undergo significant maturation during puberty and are implicated in the cause of disordered eating.[44,45,55,56] For example, estrogen is involved in the regulation of brain reward systems, such as dopaminergic and opioidergic pathways.[45,46] These systems have been consistently linked to binge eating and the consumption of palatable and sweet foods in both humans and animals.[57] Similarly, estrogen regulates the transcription of genes associated with the serotonergic system[44,55] and brain-derived neurotrophic factor.[58,59] These neurotransmitter/neurotrophin systems are involved in mood, appetite, and body weight regulation[5] and have been shown to be associated with eating disorders in neuroimaging and genetic research.[44,55,58–60] To date, no studies have directly examined changes in estrogen, genetic effects on disordered eating, and alterations in these systems or brain structures and functions during puberty.

More studies are also needed to examine mechanisms through which genetic factors influence disordered eating in males. Emerging evidence shows that adrenarche may be a critical developmental period when genetic effects increase in boys, potentially due to increasing levels of androgens. However, studies on genetic influence in boys before, during, and after puberty are still relatively sparse. Replications of existing findings are warranted, and more data are clearly required to further establish a role for androgens in disordered eating in males.

Finally, a concerning feature of the literature on the role of estrogen in disordered eating is that many studies were conducted by only our research group.[6] Despite our best efforts to include strong control conditions, test covariates, and incorporate longitudinal designs, independent replications of our findings from other laboratories are critical in order to replicate findings and confirm a role for ovarian hormones in risk for disordered eating during puberty.

CLINICAL IMPLICATIONS

Eating disorders have profound medical and psychological consequences that can be extremely disruptive to developmental processes of adolescence and young adulthood. Although sociocultural and psychological influences clearly contribute to the development of eating disorders, greater understanding of developmental shifts in genetic risk and the interplay between biological and environmental impact on eating disorders has important implications for prevention, detection, and intervention.

Prevention could be enhanced by identifying developmental windows of increased psychosocial and biological risk for developing eating disorders and targeting individuals with high genetic (eg, first-degree relatives of people with a history of disordered eating) and/or hormonal (eg, low levels of estrogen) risk during these periods. Prevention efforts could also function via psychoeducation and intervention for parents with an eating disorder or another closely related condition. Education for adolescents and their parents should include information regarding potential risks of dieting, especially during the pubertal period. Extreme dieting may forestall pubertal development, which may lead to alterations in brain development that permanently increase the risk for disordered eating. Besides refraining from extreme dieting, understanding one's potential biological sensitivity to other environmental and psychosocial risk factors may help individuals and their families attend to and manage these risks, building a more protective environment against disordered eating.

In terms of intervention, individuals with eating disorders and their families may benefit from learning about a more integrated etiologic model of these disorders, which includes discussion of biological/genetic risk in addition to psychosocial and environmental factors. Self-stigma frequently stops people in need of help from seeking treatment[61] and may elevate the shame that already affects many individuals with eating disorders.[62] A genetic and hormonal reframing of mechanisms of eating disorders may reduce this guilt and shame.[63] Understanding the biological factors involved in eating disorders may also reduce self-blame and foster empathy in caregivers. In addition, more accurate knowledge about the cause of eating disorders among the general population may reduce social stigma against those who suffer from these conditions and may in turn reduce their social isolation and psychological distress.[64]

It should be cautioned, however, that biological explanations of psychiatric conditions can sometimes exacerbate stigmatizing views by making people think that the illness is untreatable.[65] When delivering education about genetic or biological contributions to eating disorders, it should be made clear that recovery can be achieved despite the presence of biological risk. Environmental or psychosocial factors can also exacerbate underlying biological vulnerability, necessitating an integrated biopsychosocial framework for understanding and treating eating disorders.

SUMMARY

Puberty is a key developmental period during which incidence of eating disorders and their symptoms significantly increase, especially among girls.[6] Past theories have focused heavily on psychosocial factors to explain this female predominance,[4] but new evidence has transformed this understanding by showing that factors contributing to eating disorders encompass both biological and psychosocial influences. Existing research suggests that lower levels of estradiol during puberty may contribute to pubertal increases in genetic influences on disordered eating in girls.[6] Indeed, data thus far suggest that differential exposure to estrogen during puberty may result in different responsiveness to the protective influence of estrogen during puberty and into adulthood.[6,7] Although replications of existing results are needed and additional data are required to refine the model of hormonal and genetic mechanisms underlying disordered eating, those with eating disorders or who are at elevated risk may benefit from learning about genetic contributions, understanding their potential vulnerabilities, and optimizing their surrounding environment to be more protective.

REFERENCES

1. Klump KL. Puberty as a critical risk period for eating disorders: a review of human and animal studies. Horm Behav 2013;64(2):399–410.
2. Sands R, Tricker J, Sherman C, et al. Disordered eating patterns, body image, self-esteem, and physical activity in preadolescent school children. Int J Eat Disord 1997;21(2):159–66.
3. American Psychiatric Association. Diagnostic and statistical manual of mental disorders. 5th edition. Arlington (VA): American Psychiatric Publishing; 2013.
4. Fornari V, Dancyger IF. Psychosexual development and eating disorders. Adolesc Med 2003;14(1):61–75.
5. Trace SE, Baker JH, Peñas-Lledó E, et al. The genetics of eating disorders. Annu Rev Clin Psychol 2013;9:589–620.

6. Klump KL, Culbert KM, Sisk CL. Sex differences in binge eating: gonadal hormone effects across development. Annu Rev Clin Psychol 2017;13:183–207.

7. Klump KL, Fowler N, Mayhall L, et al. Estrogen moderates genetic influences on binge eating during puberty: disruption of normative processes? J Abnorm Psychol 2018;127(5):458–70.

8. Lantzouni E, Frank GR, Golden NH, et al. Reversibility of growth stunting in early onset anorexia nervosa: a prospective study. J Adolesc Health 2002;31(2):162–5.

9. Rozé C, Doyen C, Le Heuzey MF, et al. Predictors of late menarche and adult height in children with anorexia nervosa. Clin Endocrinol (Oxf) 2007;67(3):462–7.

10. Strober M, Freeman R, Lampert C, et al. Controlled family study of anorexia nervosa and bulimia nervosa: evidence of shared liability and transmission of partial syndromes. Am J Psychiatry 2000;157(3):393–401.

11. Eckert ED, Halmi KA, Marchi P, et al. Ten-year follow-up of anorexia nervosa: clinical course and outcome. Psychol Med 1995;25(1):143–56.

12. Schmidt U, Tiller J, Treasure J. Setting the scene for eating disorders: childhood care, classification and course of illness. Psychol Med 1993;23(3):663–72.

13. Walters EE, Kendler KS. Anorexia nervosa and anorexic-like syndromes in a population-based female twin sample. Am J Psychiatry 1995;152(1):64–71.

14. Luo X, Donnellan MB, Burt SA, et al. The dimensional nature of eating pathology: evidence from a direct comparison of categorical, dimensional and hybrid models. J Abnorm Psychol 2016;125(5):715–26.

15. Fonseca H, Matos MG. Are adolescent weight-related problems and general well-being essentially an issue of age, gender or rather a pubertal timing issue? J Pediatr Endocrinol Metab 2011;24(5–6):251–6.

16. Klump KL, Suisman JL, Culbert KM, et al. Binge eating proneness emerges during puberty in female rats: a longitudinal study. J Abnorm Psychol 2011;120(4):948–55.

17. Culbert KM, Sinclair EB, Hildebrandt BA, et al. Perinatal testosterone contributes to mid-to-post pubertal sex differences in risk for binge eating in male and female rats. J Abnorm Psychol 2018;127(2):239–50.

18. Culbert KM, Burt SA, Klump KL. Expanding the developmental boundaries of etiologic effects: the role of adrenarche in genetic influences on disordered eating in males. J Abnorm Psychol 2017;126(5):593–606.

19. Culbert KM, Racine SE, Klump KL. Research review: what we have learned about the causes of eating disorders - a synthesis of sociocultural, psychological, and biological research. J Child Psychol Psychiatry 2015;56(11):1141–64.

20. Klump KL, Culbert KM, Slane JD, et al. The effects of puberty on genetic risk for disordered eating: evidence for a sex difference. Psychol Med 2012;42(3):627–37.

21. Ullsperger JM, Nikolas MA. A meta-analytic review of the association between pubertal timing and psychopathology in adolescence: are there sex differences in risk? Psychol Bull 2017;143(9):903–38.

22. Klump KL, Suisman JL, Burt SA, et al. Genetic and environmental influences on disordered eating: an adoption study. J Abnorm Psychol 2009;118(4):797–805.

23. Mazzeo SE, Slof-Op't Landt MCT, van Furth EF, et al. Genetics of eating disorders: part 2. In: Wonderlich S, Mitchell J, Zwaan M de, et al, editors. Annual review of eating disorders. Oxford (England): Radcliffe Publishing Ltd; 2006. p. 17–33.

24. Suisman JL, Burt SA, McGue M, et al. Parental divorce and disordered eating: an investigation of a gene-environment interaction. Int J Eat Disord 2011;44(2):169–77.

25. Klump KL, Burt SA, Mcgue M, et al. Changes in genetic and environmental influences on disordered eating across adolescence. Arch Gen Psychiatry 2007; 64(12):1409–15.
26. Klump KL, Burt SA, Spanos A, et al. Age differences in genetic and environmental influences on weight and shape concerns. Int J Eat Disord 2010;43(8):679–88.
27. Haworth CMA, Wright MJ, Luciano M, et al. The heritability of general cognitive ability increases linearly from childhood to young adulthood. Mol Psychiatry 2010;15(11):1112–20.
28. Bouchard TJ. The Wilson effect: the increase in heritability of IQ with age. Twin Res Hum Genet 2013;16(5):923–30.
29. Turkheimer E, Haley A, Waldron M, et al. Socioeconomic status modifies heritability of IQ. Psychol Sci 2003;14(6):623–9.
30. Klump KL, McGue M, Iacono WG. Age differences in genetic and environmental influences on eating attitudes and behaviors in preadolescent and adolescent female twins. J Abnorm Psychol 2000;109(2):239–51.
31. Fairweather-Schmidt AK, Wade TD. Changes in genetic and environmental influences on disordered eating between early and late adolescence: a longitudinal twin study. Psychol Med 2015;45(15):3249–58.
32. Wade TD, Hansell NK, Crosby RD, et al. A study of changes in genetic and environmental influences on weight and shape concern across adolescence. J Abnorm Psychol 2013;122(1):119–30.
33. Parent AS, Teilmann G, Juul A, et al. The timing of normal puberty and the age limits of sexual precocity: variations around the world, secular trends, and changes after migration. Endocr Rev 2003;24(5):668–93.
34. Klump KL, McGue M, Iacono WG. Differential heritability of eating attitudes and behaviors in prepubertal versus pubertal twins. Int J Eat Disord 2003;33(3): 287–92.
35. Culbert KM, Burt SA, McGue M, et al. Puberty and the genetic diathesis of disordered eating attitudes and behaviors. J Abnorm Psychol 2009;118(4):788–96.
36. Klump KL, Perkins PS, Burt SA, et al. Puberty moderates genetic influences on disordered eating. Psychol Med 2007;37(5):627–34.
37. Klump KL, Culbert KM, O'Connor S, et al. The significant effects of puberty on the genetic diathesis of binge eating in girls. Int J Eat Disord 2017;50(8):984–9.
38. Rowe R, Pickles A, Simonoff E, et al. Bulimic symptoms in the Virginia twin study of adolescent behavioral development: correlates, comorbidity, and genetics. Biol Psychiatry 2002;51(2):172–82.
39. Baker JH, Thornton LM, Bulik CM, et al. Shared genetic effects between age at menarche and disordered eating. J Adolesc Health 2012;51(5):491–6.
40. Harden KP, Mendle J, Kretsch N. Environmental and genetic pathways between early pubertal timing and dieting in adolescence: distinguishing between objective and subjective timing. Psychol Med 2012;42(1):183–93.
41. Klump KL, Keel PK, Sisk C, et al. Preliminary evidence that estradiol moderates genetic influences on disordered eating attitudes and behaviors during puberty. Psychol Med 2010;40(10):1745–53.
42. Wilson JD, Foster DW, Kronenberg HM, et al. Williams textbook of endocrinology. 9th edition. Philadelphia: W.B. Saunders Company; 1998.
43. Klump KL, O'Connor SM, Hildebrandt BA, et al. Differential effects of estrogen and progesterone on genetic and environmental risk for emotional eating in women. Clin Psychol Sci 2016;4(5):895–908.
44. Östlund H, Keller E, Hurd YL. Estrogen receptor gene expression in relation to neuropsychiatric disorders. Ann N Y Acad Sci 2003;1007(1):54–63.

45. Becker JB. Sexual differentiation of motivation: a novel mechanism? Horm Behav 2009;55(5):646–54.
46. Craft RM. Sex differences in analgesic, reinforcing, discriminative, and motoric effects of opioids. Exp Clin Psychopharmacol 2008;16(5):376–85.
47. Klump KL, Hildebrandt BA, O'Connor SM, et al. Changes in genetic risk for emotional eating across the menstrual cycle: a longitudinal study. Psychol Med 2015;45(15):3227–37.
48. Wade GN. Gonadal hormones and behavioral regulation of body weight. Physiol Behav 1972;8(3):523–34.
49. Yu Z, Geary N, Corwin RL. Ovarian hormones inhibit fat intake under binge-type conditions in ovariectomized rats. Physiol Behav 2008;95(3):501–7.
50. Arnold AP. The organizational-activational hypothesis as the foundation for a unified theory of sexual differentiation of all mammalian tissues. Horm Behav 2009; 55(5):570–8.
51. Phoenix CH. Organizing action of prenatally administered testosterone propionate on the tissues mediating mating behavior in the female Guinea pig. Horm Behav 2009;55(5):566.
52. Klump KL, Keel PK, Culbert KM, et al. Ovarian hormones and binge eating: exploring associations in community samples. Psychol Med 2008;38(12): 1749–57.
53. Klump KL, Keel PK, Racine SE, et al. The interactive effects of estrogen and progesterone on changes in emotional eating across the menstrual cycle. J Abnorm Psychol 2013;122(1):131–7.
54. Racine SE, Culbert KM, Keel PK, et al. Differential associations between ovarian hormones and disordered eating symptoms across the menstrual cycle in women. Int J Eat Disord 2012;45(3):333–44.
55. Hildebrandt T, Alfano L, Tricamo M, et al. Conceptualizing the role of estrogens and serotonin in the development and maintenance of bulimia nervosa. Clin Psychol Rev 2010;30(6):655–68.
56. Young JK. Anorexia nervosa and estrogen: current status of the hypothesis. Neurosci Biobehav Rev 2010;34(8):1195–200.
57. Berridge KC. "Liking" and "wanting" food rewards: brain substrates and roles in eating disorders. Physiol Behav 2009;97(5):537–50.
58. Klump K, Culbert K. Molecular genetic studies of eating disorders: current and future directions. Curr Dir Psychol Sci 2007;16(1):37–41.
59. Rask-Andersen M, Olszewski PK, Levine AS, et al. Molecular mechanisms underlying anorexia nervosa: focus on human gene association studies and systems controlling food intake. Brain Res Rev 2010;62(2):147–64.
60. Kaye W. Neurobiology of anorexia and bulimia nervosa. Physiol Behav 2008; 94(1):121–35.
61. Hackler AH, Vogel DL, Wade NG. Attitudes toward seeking professional help for an eating disorder: the role of stigma and anticipated outcomes. J Couns Dev 2010;88:424–31.
62. Swan S, Andrews B. The relationship between shame, eating disorders and disclosure in treatment. Br J Clin Psychol 2003;42(4):367–78.
63. Easter MM. "Not all my fault": genetics, stigma, and personal responsibility for women with eating disorders. Soc Sci Med 2012;75(8):1408–16.
64. Corrigan PW, Rüsch N. Mental illness stereotypes and clinical care: do people avoid treatment because of stigma? Psychiatr Rehabil Ski 2002;6(3):312–34.
65. Hinshaw SP, Stier A. Stigma as related to mental disorders. Annu Rev Clin Psychol 2008;4(1):367–93.

The Neurobiology of Eating Disorders

Guido K.W. Frank, MD[a,b,]*, Megan E. Shott, BS[a,b], Marisa C. DeGuzman, BS, BA[c]

KEYWORDS

- Anorexia nervosa • Bulimia nervosa • Eating disorder • Brain • Imaging
- Neurobiology

KEY POINTS

- An eating disorder is a severe psychiatric illnesses with a complex biopsychosocial background.
- Brain imaging now allows study of the living human brain.
- Understanding the neurobiology of eating disorders holds promise for developing more effective treatments.
- New research enables the development of models for brain function and food avoidance.

INTRODUCTION

Anorexia nervosa (AN), bulimia nervosa (BN), binge eating disorder (BED), and avoidant or restrictive food intake disorder (ARFID) are severe psychiatric disorders.[1] The understanding of the brain has dramatically changed over the past century with the development of human in vivo brain imaging. Whereas earlier studies collected cerebrospinal fluid samples to study metabolites (eg, neurotransmitters), brain research now uses techniques such as MRI to study brain gray matter (GM) and white matter (WM) volumes, cortical thickness, and surface area. Also based on MRI, diffusion weighed imaging and diffusion tensor imaging measure water diffusion to test WM tract integrity and strength of WM connectivity between brain regions.[2] The most commonly used functional brain imaging technique is functional MRI, which measures changes in local blood flow as a proxy for brain activation.[3] PET and single-photon emission computed tomography (SPECT) use radioactive ligands to study glucose

Disclosure Statement: The authors have nothing to disclose.
[a] University of California San Diego, UCSD Eating Disorder Center, 4510 Executive Dr #315, San Diego, CA 92121, USA; [b] Rady Children's Hospital San Diego, San Diego, CA, USA; [c] Department of Psychiatry, University of Colorado Anschutz Medical Campus, School of Medicine, Children's Hospital Colorado, Gary Pavilion A036/B-130, 13123 East 16th Avenue, Aurora, CO 80045, USA
* Corresponding author. University of California San Diego, UCSD Eating Disorder Center, 4510 Executive Dr #315, San Diego, CA 92121
E-mail address: Guido.Frank@ucdenver.edu

metabolism or neurotransmitter receptor distribution. Neurobiological research in eating disorders (EDs) holds promise for developing a medical model perspective to reduce stigma and help develop better treatments.[4]

METHODS

This article provides a state-of-the-art review of current neurobiological research in EDs in children, adolescents, and young adults up to 25 years of age when brain structure has generally matured to adult levels while avoiding effects from aging or illness chronicity.[5] The US National Library of Medicine database, PubMed, was searched for brain research studies done in youth or young adults. Methodologies have greatly improved over the past 5 years. Neurobiological research that highlights current knowledge of ED neurobiology, with a particular emphasis on studies from the past 5 years, is presented.[6]

NEUROCHEMICAL STUDIES

PET imaging showed higher serotonin 1A-receptor binding in AN and BN when the participants were ill and after recovery, suggesting state-independent alterations. The serotonin 2A-receptor, in contrast, was normal in ill AN participants but lower after recovery, suggesting dynamic adaptations.[7,8] BN did not show significant dopamine D2-receptor group differences versus controls, but lower striatal dopamine release was associated with higher binge eating frequency.[9]

Hormones or neuroactive peptides, such as sex hormones or gut hormones, also affect brain response.[10] Those substances that regulate body homeostasis are often altered during the ill state of EDs, which may disturb normal food reward circuits.[10] Neuroendocrines and peptides, such as fat cell-derived leptin or ghrelin from the gastric mucosa, stimulate or dampen brain dopamine response and alterations in this system, which could further alter food approach in AN and BN.[11,12] To date, however, those hypotheses rely mostly on basic research. Cytokines, markers of inflammatory processes, have been found altered, and meta-analyses indicate a pattern of elevated tumor necrosis factor-alpha in AN, whereas the data on other cytokines are somewhat mixed, with no alterations in BN.[13,14] Whether those markers are relevant for ED illness development, maintenance or recovery remains elusive. Cytokines are elevated in obesity, but no data exist for BED or ARFID.

GRAY MATTER VOLUME AND CORTICAL THICKNESS

Earlier studies suggested that brain volume is universally reduced in AN, but brain structure studies in participants with EDs have found smaller, larger, or no differing volumes across varying brain regions versus controls.[15–17] Reduced cortical volumes in AN are related to illness severity and normalize during weight recovery.[18–23] Studies that controlled for short-term malnutrition and dehydration found larger left orbitofrontal cortex, as well as right insula volumes, in adolescents and adults with AN.[24,25]

The literature on BN is scarcer, and GM structure studies in adolescents or young adults with BED or ARFID are lacking. Mixed results in BN show either larger or normal regional GM volumes,[26,27] whereas another study found lower temporoparietal GM surface area due to lower WM.[28] Binge eating or purging frequency may reduce cortical volume or thickness.[29,30] A study that controlled for acute malnutrition and binge eating or purging found larger left orbitofrontal and insula volume but smaller bilateral caudate and putamen volumes.[25]

Those results highlight that food restriction, binge eating, and purging change brain structure. Insula and orbitofrontal cortex are important for taste perception and (food) reward valuation, and alterations could interfere with the drive to eat. Whether brain volume alterations drive ED behaviors remains unclear.[31] Future studies will test whether ARFID is associated with similar structural brain changes, as in AN, and whether BED is associated with reduced brain volume, as in obesity, or with regionally higher volume, measures as in BN.[32]

WHITE MATTER VOLUME, INTEGRITY, AND STRUCTURAL CONNECTIVITY

Similar to GM studies, there has been inconsistency with higher or lower localized or overall WM volumes in EDs.[24,25,33,34] Altered astrocyte density exhibited in an animal model of AN could be a mechanism for low WM volume in EDs due to malnutrition and dehydration.[35]

Water-diffusion MRI can be used to calculate fractional anisotropy (FA),[36] which is thought to reflect axonal integrity. Adolescent AN showed higher, lower, or no FA group differences.[37–40] Lower FA normalizes with weight restoration, and it is unclear whether FA has implications for ED behaviors.[41,42] The scarce literature on WM integrity and FA in BN indicates lower FA across widespread WM pathways across the whole brain, including lower FA between insula, orbitofrontal cortex, striatum, and hypothalamus.[43–45] Those regions are important for taste, reward, and energy homeostasis regulation, and altered WM connections could affect food intake regulation. Studies that estimated the number of WM connections found in AN and BN greater structural WM connectivity between insula, orbitofrontal cortex, and ventral striatum, consistent with AN after recovery.[43,46] Duration of illness correlated positively with fiber connectivity in AN, suggesting that the longer ED behaviors caused WM damage (FA reduction), which was compensated for during recovery by increasing fiber connectivity.[46]

FUNCTIONAL AND EFFECTIVE CONNECTIVITY

The posterior cingulate, medial prefrontal, medial temporal, and inferior parietal cortices, the so-called default mode network (DMN), is involved in interoception and self-relevant mentalizing (ie, making sense of self and other). Studies found elevated DMN connectivity in AN,[47–49] possibly driven by lower blood glucose.[50] The anterior cingulate, insula, and orbitofrontal cortex, the so-called salience network (SN), orients the organism to support food approach.[51] AN showed higher connectivity between the dorsal anterior and posterior cingulate gyrus, and BN showed stronger connectivity between the dorsal anterior cingulate and medial orbitofrontal cortex.[52,53] Higher dorsal anterior cingulate to precuneus connectivity in AN and BN correlated positively with body shape questionnaire scores, implicating brain regions at the interface of executive function and vision.[52] Other studies found greater resting functional connectivity in AN between ventral striatum and frontal cortex, implicating reward-processing and decision-making circuits.[37] Functional connectivity during food and nonfood passive picture viewing was higher in AN and BN in the insula, and in BN in the orbitofrontal cortex,[54] whereas young adults with AN showed lower SN connectivity during sugar tasting.[55] These patterns suggest dysfunctional SN functioning and maybe predisposing to food restriction. The prefrontal cortex, the so-called executive control network, showed lower connectivity and lower and higher connectivity in AN between the insula and frontal regions, suggesting imbalances between networks.[56,57]

All in all, higher and lower functional resting-state connectivity has been observed in participants with EDs compared with controls, implicating networks associated with executive function, reward processing, and perception, which supports the notion of those circuits being altered in EDs. SN alterations during the resting state could perturb a readiness to approach food, whereas elevated DMN activity could indicate an inability to come to an internal restful state.[58] Studies in ARFID and BED are lacking.[59]

Effective connectivity, the hierarchical or directional activation between brain regions, was higher in AN from the medial orbitofrontal cortex and insula to the inferior frontal gyrus,[57] and from the orbitofrontal cortex to the nucleus accumbens,[37] implicating taste-reward circuits. Two studies found that effective connectivity during sugar tasting was directed from the ventral striatum to the hypothalamus in AN and BN, whereas in controls the hypothalamus drove ventral striatal activity.[43,60] This was interpreted as a possible mechanism for top-down control in EDs to control homeostatic information and override hunger signals.

TASK-BASED FUNCTIONAL MRI STUDIES
Reward System

Food is a salient stimulus or natural reward, and reward pathways similar to substances of abuse are activated when people desire, approach, or eat food.[61] Important regions in this circuitry include the ventral striatum (receives midbrain dopaminergic input, drives motivation and reward approach), the orbitofrontal cortex (reward valuation), and the anterior cingulate (error monitoring, reward expectation).[61] Several but not all studies in the past in adolescents or young adults found altered reward system response in AN to food-related or body-related visual stimuli.[62–66] In a recent study in which participants saw positively valenced (nonfood and nonbody) pictures and were asked to regulate their emotions, ventral striatal activity correlated with body-related ruminations and negative affect in AN, suggesting that emotion regulation interacts with both ED thoughts and depressive feelings.[67] In a delay-discounting task (choosing between immediate smaller or delayed larger rewards), the AN group responded faster, and lower activation in AN in the cingulate and frontal regions indicated a more efficient control circuitry.[68] In another study, youth with AN learned better in response to punishment but associated brain-activation was similar versus controls.[69–71] Receiving stimuli unexpectedly has been associated with brain dopamine response and early evidence indicated heightened response to unexpected pleasant or unpleasant stimuli in AN.[72,73] A paradigm that has been closely associated with brain dopamine response is the prediction error model, a learning paradigm in which individuals learn to associate unconditioned taste with conditioned visual stimuli.[74] In 2 studies using monetary or taste stimuli, unexpected receipt or omission was reflected in higher insula and striatal brain response in adolescents with AN versus controls. Brain activation predicted weight gain during treatment, but short-term weight restoration was not associated with normalization of brain response.[75,76] Those studies suggested heightened dopamine-related brain response that does not easily normalize with weight recovery.[76] In summary, altered reward circuits in AN may be associated with altered learning and brain dopamine function, and traits such as sensitivity to punishment could be predisposing.[60]

In BN, negative affect positively correlated with striatal and pallidum brain response during milkshake receipt.[77] Low mood may, therefore, enhance the reward value of food stimuli in BN and trigger binge eating. Other studies showed less frontal cortical, ventral striatal, and hippocampus activation in BN, which correlated with binge or purge frequency in a task that provided monetary reward when navigating through a maze.[78,79] Therefore, altered learning, executive control, and reward brain response could be effects of both abnormal brain development and BN illness behavior.

Perception and Interoception

Self-perception of being fat while being underweight could be due to abnormal central interoception neurocircuitry or primarily driven by cognitive-emotional processes. Some studies in AN implicated the parietal and occipital cortices when viewing self or others.[80,81] Neuropsychological studies implicated altered nonvisual perception, such as haptic (tactile) perception, proprioception (sense of one's position in space), or interoception (sense of internal organs) in AN, showing altered insula response in AN.[82] This suggested that the insula may have an essential function in the intersection between interoception and cognitive-emotional processing in AN. Some studies implicated taste perception in EDs. In AN, the insula (primary taste cortex) poorly distinguished between taste stimuli.[83] In studies on binge eating, bitter taste led to higher medial prefrontal electroencephalography signal, or umami taste, more strongly activated the insula in BN, whereas hedonic ratings were lower.[84,85]

Cognition

During a reversal learning task involving positive and negative feedback, participants with AN changed behavior strategy more frequently after negative feedback, related to cingulate activation.[86] During the Wisconsin Card Sorting Test for cognitive flexibility, participants with AN had higher activation during behavior change in the frontal, parietal, and occipital regions but lower activation during learning or maintaining rule-based behavior.[87] Visual attention in participants with BN led to higher activation in parietooccipital regions but lower response in the DMN versus controls, and behavior control was associated with lower activation in the anterior cingulate.[88] Behaviorally, groups performed similarly in the studies, and the meaning of altered brain function in the context of normal behavioral response needs further study. Individuals with BN showed worse cognitive performance when food images were intermixed with the task procedures, whereas premotor cortex and dorsal striatum were more strongly activated compared with controls, suggesting a distressing effect.[84] In another study, BN showed that positive emotions improved performance on response inhibition.[89] Therefore, mood may be an important factor for recovery.

Social Function and Stress

During a self-and-other social evaluation task, anxiety and body shape concerns correlated inversely in participants with AN compared with controls, with prefrontal and cingulate brain response, implicating those regions.[90] Gentle touch or intimate visual stimuli were rated less pleasant in participants with AN compared with controls, and were associated with lower caudate or parietal activity, suggesting reduced reward experience.[91,92]

MICROBIOTA AND MICROBIOME

The human microbiota, up to 100 trillion symbiotic microbial cells, is primarily bacteria in the gut.[93] Their collective genomes are called microbiome.[94] There are well-known neural connections between gut and brain, and those organisms may affect psychiatric disorders, including EDs.[95] Various studies in participants with AN have found alterations compared with controls in microbial composition, and microbe diversity in AN may correlate with body mass index and also, for instance, blood insulin levels.[96-98] Healthy competitive athletes had the highest number of microbiota species compared with ED and control groups, significantly higher versus both AN and obese individuals. Also, dietary fiber, vitamin D, and magnesium intake correlated positively with microbiota species.[99] However, microbiota diversity also normalizes with weight recovery, and it is unclear whether microbiota could be causal for illness behavior aside from ED behaviors altering gut microbiota.[97,98,100] No studies exist in other EDs. However, BN and BED were associated with antimicrobial medication use, suggesting a role for the immune system. In summary, study of microbiota and the microbiome is an emerging field that could provide an important aspect of illness pathophysiology in EDs.

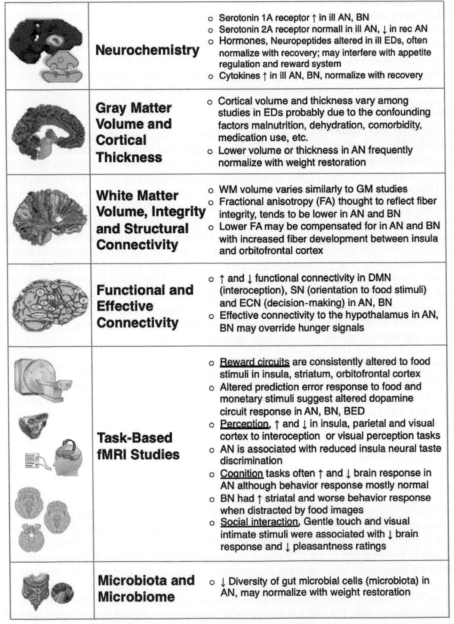

	Neurochemistry	o Serotonin 1A receptor ↑ in ill AN, BN o Serotonin 2A receptor normall in ill AN, ↓ in rec AN o Hormones, Neuropeptides altered in ill EDs, often normalize with recovery; may interfere with appetite regulation and reward system o Cytokines ↑ in ill AN, BN, normalize with recovery
	Gray Matter Volume and Cortical Thickness	o Cortical volume and thickness vary among studies in EDs probably due to the confounding factors malnutrition, dehydration, comorbidity, medication use, etc. o Lower volume or thickness in AN frequently normalize with weight restoration
	White Matter Volume, Integrity and Structural Connectivity	o WM volume varies similarly to GM studies o Fractional anisotropy (FA) thought to reflect fiber integrity, tends to be lower in AN and BN o Lower FA may be compensated for in AN and BN with increased fiber development between insula and orbitofrontal cortex
	Functional and Effective Connectivity	o ↑ and ↓ functional connectivity in DMN (interoception), SN (orientation to food stimuli) and ECN (decision-making) in AN, BN o Effective connectivity to the hypothalamus in AN, BN may override hunger signals
	Task-Based fMRI Studies	o Reward circuits are consistently altered to food stimuli in insula, striatum, orbitofrontal cortex o Altered prediction error response to food and monetary stimuli suggest altered dopamine circuit response in AN, BN, BED o Perception, ↑ and ↓ in insula, parietal and visual cortex to interoception or visual perception tasks o AN is associated with reduced insula neural taste discrimination o Cognition tasks often ↑ and ↓ brain response in AN although behavior response mostly normal o BN had ↑ striatal and worse behavior response when distracted by food images o Social interaction, Gentle touch and visual intimate stimuli were associated with ↓ brain response and ↓ pleasantness ratings
	Microbiota and Microbiome	o ↓ Diversity of gut microbial cells (microbiota) in AN, may normalize with weight restoration

Fig. 1. Summary of neurobiological findings in eating disorders. ↓, decreased; ↑, increased; ECN, executive control network; fMRI, functional MRI; rec, recovered.

SUMMARY

This article summarizes current knowledge on the neurobiology of eating disorders (**Fig. 1**). Although this field has grown significantly over the past decade, it is still small overall and the studies available often have low participant numbers, limiting power and study reliability, and many results have not been replicated. The authors argue for rigorous well-powered studies to find consensus across research laboratories to identify treatment targets for EDs.[101] Another critical issue is that BED, especially ARFID, is mostly an unexplored area of neurobiological research. Nevertheless, the body of research in EDs identified the importance of the short-term impact of ED behaviors, especially on brain structure, and brain reward pathways are most consistently implicated in altered brain activity across EDs. The latter is a promising target for treatment development.

ACKNOWLEDGMENTS

This work was supported by National Institute of Mental Health grants MH096777 and MH103436 (both to G.K.W. Frank). The funders had no role in study design, data collection or analysis, decision to publish, or preparation of the article.

REFERENCES

1. American Psychiatric Association. Desk reference to the diagnostic criteria from DSM-5. Washington, DC: American Psychiatric Publishing; 2013.
2. Filler A. Magnetic resonance neurography and diffusion tensor imaging: origins, history, and clinical impact of the first 50,000 cases with an assessment of efficacy and utility in a prospective 5000-patient study group. Neurosurgery 2009; 65(4 Suppl):A29–43.
3. Raichle ME. Behind the scenes of functional brain imaging: a historical and physiological perspective. Proc Natl Acad Sci U S A 1998;95(3):765–72.
4. Vengeliene V, Bespalov A, Rossmanith M, et al. Towards trans-diagnostic mechanisms in psychiatry: neurobehavioral profile of rats with a loss-of-function point mutation in the dopamine transporter gene. Dis Model Mech 2017;10(4): 451–61.
5. Shaw P, Kabani NJ, Lerch JP, et al. Neurodevelopmental trajectories of the human cerebral cortex. J Neurosci 2008;28(14):3586–94.
6. Poldrack RA, Baker CI, Durnez J, et al. Scanning the horizon: towards transparent and reproducible neuroimaging research. Nat Rev Neurosci 2017; 18(2):115–26.
7. Frank GK. Advances from neuroimaging studies in eating disorders. CNS Spectr 2015;20:391–400.
8. Frank GK. The perfect storm - a bio-psycho-social risk model for developing and maintaining eating disorders. Front Behav Neurosci 2016;10:44.
9. Broft A, Shingleton R, Kaufman J, et al. Striatal dopamine in bulimia nervosa: a PET imaging study. Int J Eat Disord 2012;45(5):648–56.
10. Monteleone P, Maj M. Dysfunctions of leptin, ghrelin, BDNF and endocannabinoids in eating disorders: beyond the homeostatic control of food intake. Psychoneuroendocrinology 2013;38(3):312–30.
11. Berner LA, Brown TA, Lavender JM, et al. Neuroendocrinology of reward in anorexia nervosa and bulimia nervosa: beyond leptin and ghrelin. Mol Cell Endocrinol 2018 [pii:S0303-7207(18)30313-7].

12. Monteleone AM, Castellini G, Volpe U, et al. Neuroendocrinology and brain imaging of reward in eating disorders: a possible key to the treatment of anorexia nervosa and bulimia nervosa. Prog Neuropsychopharmacol Biol Psychiatry 2018;80(Pt B):132–42.

13. Solmi M, Veronese N, Favaro A, et al. Inflammatory cytokines and anorexia nervosa: a meta-analysis of cross-sectional and longitudinal studies. Psychoneuroendocrinology 2015;51:237–52.

14. Dalton B, Whitmore V, Patsalos O, et al. A systematic review of in vitro cytokine production in eating disorders. Mol Cell Endocrinol 2018 [pii:S0303-7207(18) 30287-9].

15. Van den Eynde F, Suda M, Broadbent H, et al. Structural magnetic resonance imaging in eating disorders: a systematic review of voxel-based morphometry studies. Eur Eat Disord Rev 2012;20(2):94–105.

16. Donnelly B, Touyz S, Hay P, et al. Neuroimaging in bulimia nervosa and binge eating disorder: a systematic review. J Eat Disord 2018;6:3.

17. Frank GK. What causes eating disorders, and what do they cause? Biol Psychiatry 2015;77(7):602–3.

18. King JA, Geisler D, Ritschel F, et al. Global cortical thinning in acute anorexia nervosa normalizes following long-term weight restoration. Biol Psychiatry 2015;77(7):624–32.

19. Bernardoni F, King JA, Geisler D, et al. Weight restoration therapy rapidly reverses cortical thinning in anorexia nervosa: a longitudinal study. Neuroimage 2016;130:214–22.

20. Solstrand Dahlberg L, Wiemerslage L, Swenne I, et al. Adolescents newly diagnosed with eating disorders have structural differences in brain regions linked with eating disorder symptoms. Nord J Psychiatry 2017;71(3):188–96.

21. Martin Monzon B, Henderson LA, Madden S, et al. Grey matter volume in adolescents with anorexia nervosa and associated eating disorder symptoms. Eur J Neurosci 2017;46(7):2297–307.

22. Kohmura K, Adachi Y, Tanaka S, et al. Regional decrease in gray matter volume is related to body dissatisfaction in anorexia nervosa. Psychiatry Res Neuroimaging 2017;267:51–8.

23. Nickel K, Joos A, Tebartz van Elst L, et al. Recovery of cortical volume and thickness after remission from acute anorexia nervosa. Int J Eat Disord 2018;51(9): 1056–69.

24. Frank GK, Shott ME, Hagman JO, et al. Localized brain volume and white matter integrity alterations in adolescent anorexia nervosa. J Am Acad Child Adolesc Psychiatry 2013;52(10):1066–75.e5.

25. Frank GK, Shott ME, Hagman JO, et al. Alterations in brain structures related to taste reward circuitry in ill and recovered anorexia nervosa and in bulimia nervosa. Am J Psychiatry 2013;170(10):1152–60.

26. Amianto F, Caroppo P, D'Agata F, et al. Brain volumetric abnormalities in patients with anorexia and bulimia nervosa: a voxel-based morphometry study. Psychiatry Res 2013;213(3):210–6.

27. Joos A, Kloppel S, Hartmann A, et al. Voxel-based morphometry in eating disorders: correlation of psychopathology with grey matter volume. Psychiatry Res 2010;182(2):146–51.

28. Marsh R, Stefan M, Bansal R, et al. Anatomical characteristics of the cerebral surface in bulimia nervosa. Biol Psychiatry 2015;77(7):616–23.

29. Berner LA, Stefan M, Lee S, et al. Altered cortical thickness and attentional deficits in adolescent girls and women with bulimia nervosa. J Psychiatry Neurosci 2018;43(3):151–60.

30. Westwater ML, Seidlitz J, Diederen KMJ, et al. Associations between cortical thickness, structural connectivity and severity of dimensional bulimia nervosa symptomatology. Psychiatry Res Neuroimaging 2018;271:118–25.

31. King JA, Frank GKW, Thompson PM, et al. Structural neuroimaging of anorexia nervosa: future directions in the quest for mechanisms underlying dynamic alterations. Biol Psychiatry 2018;83(3):224–34.

32. Riederer JW, Shott ME, Deguzman M, et al. Understanding neuronal architecture in obesity through analysis of white matter connection strength. Front Hum Neurosci 2016;10:271.

33. Lazaro L, Andres S, Calvo A, et al. Normal gray and white matter volume after weight restoration in adolescents with anorexia nervosa. Int J Eat Disord 2013;46(8):841–8.

34. Seitz J, Herpertz-Dahlmann B, Konrad K. Brain morphological changes in adolescent and adult patients with anorexia nervosa. J Neural Transm (Vienna) 2016;123(8):949–59.

35. Frintrop L, Liesbrock J, Paulukat L, et al. Reduced astrocyte density underlying brain volume reduction in activity-based anorexia rats. World J Biol Psychiatry 2018;19(3):225–35.

36. Huisman TA. Diffusion-weighted and diffusion tensor imaging of the brain, made easy. Cancer Imaging 2010;10 Spec no A:S163–71.

37. Cha J, Ide JS, Bowman FD, et al. Abnormal reward circuitry in anorexia nervosa: a longitudinal, multimodal MRI study. Hum Brain Mapp 2016;37(11):3835–46.

38. Pfuhl G, King JA, Geisler D, et al. Preserved white matter microstructure in young patients with anorexia nervosa? Hum Brain Mapp 2016;37(11):4069–83.

39. Travis KE, Golden NH, Feldman HM, et al. Abnormal white matter properties in adolescent girls with anorexia nervosa. Neuroimage Clin 2015;9:648–59.

40. Vogel K, Timmers I, Kumar V, et al. White matter microstructural changes in adolescent anorexia nervosa including an exploratory longitudinal study. Neuroimage Clin 2016;11:614–21.

41. Phillipou A, Carruthers SP, Di Biase MA, et al. White matter microstructure in anorexia nervosa. Hum Brain Mapp 2018;39(11):4385–92.

42. von Schwanenflug N, Muller DK, King JA, et al. Dynamic changes in white matter microstructure in anorexia nervosa: findings from a longitudinal study. Psychol Med 2019;49(9):1555–64.

43. Frank GK, Shott ME, Riederer J, et al. Altered structural and effective connectivity in anorexia and bulimia nervosa in circuits that regulate energy and reward homeostasis. Transl Psychiatry 2016;6(11):e932.

44. Mettler LN, Shott ME, Pryor T, et al. White matter integrity is reduced in bulimia nervosa. Int J Eat Disord 2013;46(3):264–73.

45. He X, Stefan M, Terranova K, et al. Altered white matter microstructure in adolescents and adults with bulimia nervosa. Neuropsychopharmacology 2016;41(7):1841–8.

46. Shott ME, Pryor TL, Yang TT, et al. Greater insula white matter fiber connectivity in women recovered from anorexia nervosa. Neuropsychopharmacology 2016;41(2):498–507.

47. Cowdrey FA, Filippini N, Park RJ, et al. Increased resting state functional connectivity in the default mode network in recovered anorexia nervosa. Hum Brain Mapp 2014;35(2):483–91.

48. Boehm I, Geisler D, King JA, et al. Increased resting state functional connectivity in the fronto-parietal and default mode network in anorexia nervosa. Front Behav Neurosci 2014;8:346.

49. Boehm I, Geisler D, Tam F, et al. Partially restored resting-state functional connectivity in women recovered from anorexia nervosa. J Psychiatry Neurosci 2016;41(6):377–85.

50. Ishibashi K, Sakurai K, Shimoji K, et al. Altered functional connectivity of the default mode network by glucose loading in young, healthy participants. BMC Neurosci 2018;19(1):33.

51. Seeley WW, Menon V, Schatzberg AF, et al. Dissociable intrinsic connectivity networks for salience processing and executive control. J Neurosci 2007; 27(9):2349–56.

52. Lee S, Ran Kim K, Ku J, et al. Resting-state synchrony between anterior cingulate cortex and precuneus relates to body shape concern in anorexia nervosa and bulimia nervosa. Psychiatry Res 2014;221(1):43–8.

53. Biezonski D, Cha J, Steinglass J, et al. Evidence for thalamocortical circuit abnormalities and associated cognitive dysfunctions in underweight individuals with anorexia nervosa. Neuropsychopharmacology 2016;41(6):1560–8.

54. Kim KR, Ku J, Lee JH, et al. Functional and effective connectivity of anterior insula in anorexia nervosa and bulimia nervosa. Neurosci Lett 2012;521(2):152–7.

55. McFadden KL, Tregellas JR, Shott ME, et al. Reduced salience and default mode network activity in women with anorexia nervosa. J Psychiatry Neurosci 2014;39(3):178–88.

56. Gaudio S, Piervincenzi C, Beomonte Zobel B, et al. Altered resting-state functional connectivity of anterior cingulate cortex in drug-naive adolescents at the earliest stages of anorexia nervosa. Sci Rep 2015;5:10818.

57. Kullmann S, Giel KE, Teufel M, et al. Aberrant network integrity of the inferior frontal cortex in women with anorexia nervosa. Neuroimage Clin 2014;4:615–22.

58. Raichle ME. The brain's default mode network. Annu Rev Neurosci 2015;38: 433–47.

59. Heine L, Soddu A, Gomez F, et al. Resting state networks and consciousness: alterations of multiple resting state network connectivity in physiological, pharmacological, and pathological consciousness States. Front Psychol 2012;3:295.

60. Frank GKW, DeGuzman MC, Shott ME, et al. Association of brain reward learning response with harm avoidance, weight gain, and hypothalamic effective connectivity in adolescent anorexia nervosa. JAMA Psychiatry 2018; 75(10):1071–80.

61. Kelley AE, Berridge KC. The neuroscience of natural rewards: relevance to addictive drugs. J Neurosci 2002;22(9):3306–11.

62. Fladung AK, Gron G, Grammer K, et al. A neural signature of anorexia nervosa in the ventral striatal reward system. Am J Psychiatry 2010;167(2):206–12.

63. Holsen LM, Lawson EA, Blum J, et al. Food motivation circuitry hypoactivation related to hedonic and nonhedonic aspects of hunger and satiety in women with active anorexia nervosa and weight-restored women with anorexia nervosa. J Psychiatry Neurosci 2012;37(5):322–32.

64. Sanders N, Smeets PA, van Elburg AA, et al. Altered food-cue processing in chronically ill and recovered women with anorexia nervosa. Front Behav Neurosci 2015;9:46.

65. Horndasch S, Roesch J, Forster C, et al. Neural processing of food and emotional stimuli in adolescent and adult anorexia nervosa patients. PLoS One 2018;13(3):e0191059.

66. Boehm I, King JA, Bernardoni F, et al. Subliminal and supraliminal processing of reward-related stimuli in anorexia nervosa. Psychol Med 2018;48(5):790–800.

67. Seidel M, King JA, Ritschel F, et al. The real-life costs of emotion regulation in anorexia nervosa: a combined ecological momentary assessment and fMRI study. Transl Psychiatry 2018;8(1):28.

68. King JA, Geisler D, Bernardoni F, et al. Altered neural efficiency of decision making during temporal reward discounting in anorexia nervosa. J Am Acad Child Adolesc Psychiatry 2016;55(11):972–9.

69. Bischoff-Grethe A, McCurdy D, Grenesko-Stevens E, et al. Altered brain response to reward and punishment in adolescents with anorexia nervosa. Psychiatry Res Neuroimaging 2013;214(3):331–40.

70. Bernardoni F, Geisler D, King JA, et al. Altered medial frontal feedback learning signals in anorexia nervosa. Biol Psychiatry 2018;83(3):235–43.

71. Foerde K, Steinglass JE. Decreased feedback learning in anorexia nervosa persists after weight restoration. Int J Eat Disord 2017;50(4):415–23.

72. Cowdrey FA, Park RJ, Harmer CJ, et al. Increased neural processing of rewarding and aversive food stimuli in recovered anorexia nervosa. Biol Psychiatry 2011;70(8):736–43.

73. Schultz W. Getting formal with dopamine and reward. Neuron 2002;36(2):241–63.

74. O'Doherty JP, Dayan P, Friston K, et al. Temporal difference models and reward-related learning in the human brain. Neuron 2003;38(2):329–37.

75. DeGuzman M, Shott ME, Yang TT, et al. Association of elevated reward prediction error response with weight gain in adolescent anorexia nervosa. Am J Psychiatry 2017;174(6):557–65.

76. Frank GK, Shott ME, Hagman JO, et al. The partial dopamine D2 receptor agonist aripiprazole is associated with weight gain in adolescent anorexia nervosa. Int J Eat Disord 2017;50(4):447–50.

77. Bohon C, Stice E. Negative affect and neural response to palatable food intake in bulimia nervosa. Appetite 2012;58(3):964–70.

78. Cyr M, Wang Z, Tau GZ, et al. Reward-based spatial learning in teens with bulimia nervosa. J Am Acad Child Adolesc Psychiatry 2016;55(11):962–71.e3.

79. Frank GK. Altered brain reward circuits in eating disorders: chicken or egg? Curr Psychiatry Rep 2013;15(10):396.

80. Phillipou A, Abel LA, Castle DJ, et al. Self perception and facial emotion perception of others in anorexia nervosa. Front Psychol 2015;6:1181.

81. Fonville L, Giampietro V, Surguladze S, et al. Increased BOLD signal in the fusiform gyrus during implicit emotion processing in anorexia nervosa. Neuroimage Clin 2014;4:266–73.

82. Kerr KL, Moseman SE, Avery JA, et al. Altered insula activity during visceral interoception in weight-restored patients with anorexia nervosa. Neuropsychopharmacology 2016;41(2):521–8.

83. Frank GK, Shott ME, Keffler C, et al. Extremes of eating are associated with reduced neural taste discrimination. Int J Eat Disord 2016;49(6):603–12.

84. Lee JE, Namkoong K, Jung YC. Impaired prefrontal cognitive control over interference by food images in binge-eating disorder and bulimia nervosa. Neurosci Lett 2017;651:95–101.

85. Setsu R, Hirano Y, Tokunaga M, et al. Increased subjective distaste and altered insula activity to umami tastant in patients with bulimia nervosa. Front Psychiatry 2017;8:172.

86. Geisler D, Ritschel F, King JA, et al. Increased anterior cingulate cortex response precedes behavioural adaptation in anorexia nervosa. Sci Rep 2017;7:42066.
87. Lao-Kaim NP, Fonville L, Giampietro VP, et al. Aberrant function of learning and cognitive control networks underlie inefficient cognitive flexibility in anorexia nervosa: a cross-sectional fMRI study. PLoS One 2015;10(5):e0124027.
88. Seitz J, Hueck M, Dahmen B, et al. Attention network dysfunction in bulimia nervosa - an fMRI study. PLoS One 2016;11(9):e0161329.
89. Dreyfuss MFW, Riegel ML, Pedersen GA, et al. Patients with bulimia nervosa do not show typical neurodevelopment of cognitive control under emotional influences. Psychiatry Res Neuroimaging 2017;266:59–65.
90. Xu J, Harper JA, Van Enkevort EA, et al. Neural activations are related to body-shape, anxiety, and outcomes in adolescent anorexia nervosa. J Psychiatr Res 2017;87:1–7.
91. Davidovic M, Karjalainen L, Starck G, et al. Abnormal brain processing of gentle touch in anorexia nervosa. Psychiatry Res Neuroimaging 2018;281:53–60.
92. van Zutphen L, Maier S, Siep N, et al. Intimate stimuli result in fronto-parietal activation changes in anorexia nervosa. Eat Weight Disord 2018. [Epub ahead of print].
93. Ursell LK, Metcalf JL, Parfrey LW, et al. Defining the human microbiome. Nutr Rev 2012;70(Suppl 1):S38–44.
94. Turnbaugh PJ, Ley RE, Hamady M, et al. The human microbiome project. Nature 2007;449(7164):804–10.
95. Weltens N, Iven J, Van Oudenhove L, et al. The gut-brain axis in health neuroscience: implications for functional gastrointestinal disorders and appetite regulation. Ann N Y Acad Sci 2018;1428(1):129–50.
96. Borgo F, Riva A, Benetti A, et al. Microbiota in anorexia nervosa: the triangle between bacterial species, metabolites and psychological tests. PLoS One 2017; 12(6):e0179739.
97. Schwensen HF, Kan C, Treasure J, et al. A systematic review of studies on the faecal microbiota in anorexia nervosa: future research may need to include microbiota from the small intestine. Eat Weight Disord 2018;23(4):399–418.
98. Kleiman SC, Watson HJ, Bulik-Sullivan EC, et al. The intestinal microbiota in acute anorexia nervosa and during renourishment: relationship to depression, anxiety, and eating disorder psychopathology. Psychosom Med 2015;77(9): 969–81.
99. Morkl S, Lackner S, Muller W, et al. Gut microbiota and body composition in anorexia nervosa inpatients in comparison to athletes, overweight, obese, and normal weight controls. Int J Eat Disord 2017;50(12):1421–31.
100. Mack I, Penders J, Cook J, et al. Is the impact of starvation on the gut microbiota specific or unspecific to anorexia nervosa? A narrative review based on a systematic literature search. Curr Neuropharmacol 2018;16(8):1131–49.
101. Frank GKW, Favaro A, Marsh R, et al. Toward valid and reliable brain imaging results in eating disorders. Int J Eat Disord 2018;51(3):250–61.

Eating Disorders in Males

Sasha Gorrell, PhD, Stuart B. Murray, PhD*

KEYWORDS

- Eating disorders • Male eating disorders • Anorexia nervosa • Bulimia nervosa
- Binge eating disorder • Muscle dysmorphia

KEY POINTS

- Eating disorders occur among a significant minority of youth and adolescent males.
- Eating disorder symptom presentation and risk factors are specific to males, particularly related to body image concerns.
- Future study of adolescent males must test screening and assessment measures for use among male populations.
- Precision screening and treatment efforts are critical in appropriately addressing eating disorders among youth and adolescent males.

INTRODUCTION AND HISTORICAL CONTEXT

Eating disorders (EDs) are pernicious psychiatric illnesses associated with significant psychiatric and medical morbidity and mortality, and at significant personal, familial, and societal costs.[1] Historically, EDs are among the most gendered of psychiatric illnesses, and it was not until nearly a century after anorexia nervosa (AN) was first clinically described[2] that the notion of male ED presentation was broached in the extant literature.[3] Particularly as amenorrhea, historically a hallmark feature of AN, does not have a direct endocrine equivalent in male patients, most twentieth century literature does not recognize the disorder if not among females. This notion eventually gave way to the realization that males account for a substantial number of cases, with more recent evidence suggesting that males comprise approximately 1 in 4 presentations of bulimia nervosa (BN) and AN.[4] Thus, it is no longer tenable to suggest that EDs are relatively uncommon among males, or to assume that males account for a negligible proportion of the public health burden associated with EDs. However, as an unfortunate consequence of historical inattention, the way in which EDs are assessed and treated is largely reflective of a female-oriented diagnostic framework. Further, less than 1% of current peer-reviewed, published articles relate specifically to male

Disclosure Statement: The authors have no commercial relationships to disclose.
Department of Psychiatry, University of California, San Francisco, 401 Parnassus Avenue, San Francisco, CA 94143, USA
* Corresponding author.
E-mail address: stuart.murray@ucsf.edu

Child Adolesc Psychiatric Clin N Am 28 (2019) 641–651
https://doi.org/10.1016/j.chc.2019.05.012
1056-4993/19/© 2019 Elsevier Inc. All rights reserved.

presentation of AN,[5] resulting in a conceptualization of the clinical profile of ED among males as largely an extrapolation of findings from female samples. This approach is predicated on the notion that the presentation of ED is similar across the sexes, although mounting evidence now suggests noteworthy differences. In the following discussion of this broad subject domain, current relevant evidence on EDs among males is synthesized, and clinical and theoretic implications are discussed along with critical directions for future research.

EPIDEMIOLOGY AND PREVALENCE RATES

It is likely that prevalence rates for male ED cited in much of the recent history of research is a gross underestimate. Emerging evidence in community settings now indicates that rates of ED in males are increasing at a faster rate than for females, and with no degree of difference in clinical severity of symptoms across the sexes.[6,7] Some population-based data suggest that there are no sex differences in the age of presentation of EDs,[8] including for early-onset (<14 years old) cases.[9] Specifically, preadolescent presentation of ED in males comprises more than 1 in 4 cases in specialty clinics in Australia[9] and as many as one-third of cases in the United Kingdom.[10] Further, ED diagnosis in non-ED settings (ie, gastroenterology) demonstrate increased rates in males, with nearly two-thirds of avoidant/restrictive food intake disorder (ARFID) diagnoses presenting among preadolescent males.[11] Recent study of male adolescents that amalgamated both full and partial EDs indicated prevalence rates of full or partial BN (0.2%), and full or partial binge eating disorder (BED) (0.4%) to be lower than in females.[12] These rates cited in adolescents are lower than in adult males, which might be reflective of some data that indicate later onset of EDs in males compared with females.[4] Some evidence suggests that later onset in males may be more specific to AN than for other EDs.[13] However, given the conflicting evidence for age of onset for ED among males, further study on prevalence is critical, particularly in population-based, primary care, and community settings.[7,14]

SIMILARITIES AND DIFFERENCES IN PRESENTATION OF EATING DISORDERS ACROSS THE SEXES

Along with the paucity of empirical research devoted solely to male populations, many full-scale clinical trials continue to exclude male patients on the premise of their assumed atypicality.[14] Although many symptoms of ED among males may indeed be qualitatively different than for females, gold standard assessments for EDs demonstrate a lack of sensitivity in detecting and qualifying ED symptoms in males.[15,16] Many EDs in males may be undetected, or at least indexed with symptoms that appear less in number or in severity. One of the hallmark features of ED, overvaluation of weight and shape, is specifically predicated on internalization of a thin ideal. The widespread screening efforts for thinness-oriented ED behaviors that support this cardinal feature (eg, caloric restriction) are largely due to researchers who must extrapolate ED symptoms from female samples. However, this assessment strategy does not take into account differences in body image among males. Specifically, the ideal body type that is typically presented among males, and henceforth potentially idealized and internalized, centers on muscularity. Subsequently, with this priority on screening for symptoms that may not directly apply to many males, lower scores are consistently reported among males in standard ED assessments.[16,17] In 1 study of adolescent high school students, only 4.9% of boys reported overvaluation of body weight or shape compared with 24.2% of girls.[18] Future studies might aid in confirming whether these findings support the notion that body image distortion in males has later onset, or if these results are instead a reflection of insufficient illness detection by focusing on the thin ideal more typical in women. In the following sections, prevalence estimates, as well as factors that are both similar and divergent across the sexes in presentation of transdiagnostic EDs, are presented.

Anorexia Nervosa

According to the latest *Diagnostic and Statistical Manual of Mental Disorders* (DSM-5), diagnostic criteria for AN consists of

1. Persistent restriction of energy intake
2. Intense fear of weight gain or becoming fat
3. Disturbance in how the body is experienced or undue influence of shape and weight on self-evaluation[19]

Criteria from DSM-IV that have since been abandoned include amenorrhea and endocrine dysfunction, which has no direct equivalent for men but might manifest in loss of sexual potency or decreased testosterone. In community-based samples, the lifetime prevalence of AN for males is estimated at 0.1% to 0.3%.[4,8,20–22] In contrast, in clinical settings, rates of AN are considerably increased, with males constituting 5% to 11% of individuals with EDs (including, but not limited to, AN) receiving specialist treatment. The discrepancy in these estimates is likely because of differences across the sexes in treatment seeking and mental health stigma that may disproportionately affect males with EDs.[7] Beyond inconsistencies in presentation for treatment, symptoms associated with AN may appear subtly different across the sexes. For example, instead of a goal of emaciation as might be commonly expressed among females with AN, dietary restriction and restraint among males with AN may be more oriented toward leanness, in the interest of enhancing muscle definition.[23] Consistent with this premise, adolescent males with AN are more likely to report a desire to have "6-pack" abdominal muscles than to have a flat stomach.[15]

Possibly a result of a lack of nuance in screening for such subtleties in symptom presentation, in a population of high school students, adolescent males reported episodes of extreme dietary restriction at least 3 times per week at a rate of 2.3%, a prevalence estimate that was considerably lower than for females (11.5%).[18] In this same sample, regular compulsive exercise (specifically motivated by a reported drive for thinness) was reported by 5.3 % of males (vs 5.4% of females), with no sex differences evident in the proportion of participants who reported this symptom. The presence of compulsive exercise, a symptom commonly expressed across EDs but particularly characteristic of AN, has been found to be similar in male and female adolescents.[20,24]

Bulimia Nervosa

Bulimia nervosa is characterized by recurrent episodes of binge eating, the use of 1 or more compensatory strategies intended to offset the impact of binge episodes, and overvaluation of weight and shape.[19] Lifetime prevalence estimates for BN among males range between 0.1% and 1.6%[4,8,20,21] with males comprising approximately one-third of all BN cases in the general population.[4,25] Compared with adult samples with BN, there is little empirical evidence of the adolescent experience of BN, and even less so among males. That said, there are some indications that male BN, similar to male AN, presents with nuanced differences in symptom presentation.

Some of these differences include that within bulimic syndrome symptoms, boys report less eating concerns and might not experience as much loss of control as females of the same age group.[18] These specific findings are reflected in lower scores for BN behaviors on standard assessment measures. However, in a large sample of adolescent boys, 6.0% of boys reported regular episodes of objective binge eating, and 8.3% reported regular episodes of loss of control eating.[18] Another behavior that is likely more common among boys specifically endorsing body image concerns related to muscularity (described in more detail later) is a phenomenon referred to as a "cheat meal." This term refers to the consumption of a large number of calories as a periodic deviation from what is customarily a muscularity-oriented dietary regimen, in a manner that specifically includes foods that are ordinarily prohibited or restricted.[5,26,27] Notably, even though these meals typically represent the number of calories that might be consumed in an objective binge episode (eg, 1000–9000 calories), they are believed to augment metabolic function to continue to achieve muscular bulk.[5,26] These cheat meals can also be accompanied by subjective loss of control, as well as compensation (eg, increased workout activity), but it remains unclear if this behavior is also associated qualitatively with distress.[26]

Binge Eating Disorder

Review of the extant adult literature indicates that binge eating seems to be the most common ED behavior in males, with a prevalence nearly equivalent to that of females among adult samples based on DSM-IV criteria.[4,7] Current DSM-5 diagnostic criteria for BED requires that objective binge eating episodes must occur with a minimum frequency of once per week for 3 months.[19] These current criteria are a reduction in frequency from DSM-IV, which required twice weekly episodes, and thus it is reasonable to conclude that the number of men with BED is systematically increased with the advent of DSM-5. Notably, a study excluding those adults who met DSM-IV criteria (ie, therefore assessing only those with a subthreshold BED presentation) found that males were 3 times as likely as females to report this frequency of binge eating.[4] Among high school adolescents, 6.0% of male students (vs 16.6% of female students) engaged in at least weekly objective binge eating over the past month.[18] Also evident in this sample, 3.4% of boys (vs 12.3% of girls) in a population-level high school survey reported at least weekly episodes of subjective binge eating.[18] Taken together, it is possible that males endorse less binge eating behavior, but future research is indicated to determine whether this report is a function of objective behavioral indices or due to nonresponse bias in reporting loss of control over eating.

Avoidant Restrictive Food Intake Disorder

ARFID, included in DSM-5 to replace the DSM-IV diagnosis of feeding disorder of infancy and early childhood, is characterized by avoidant or restrictive eating behavior resulting in 1 or more of the following:

1. Significant weight loss (or failure to achieve expected growth)
2. Nutritional deficiency
3. Dependence on oral nutritional supplements or enteral feeding, or
4. Significant interference with psychosocial functioning[19]

As restrictive eating is not associated with weight or shape concerns, screening and diagnosis of ARFID may be more equal across the sexes. Among youth and adolescents seeking treatment of an ED, approximately 14% are diagnosed with ARFID and, compared with other EDs, a larger proportion of these cases, up to 35%, are boys.[28-31] As ARFID is comparatively recent in its characterization as a pediatric ED, future research is needed to illuminate sex differences in symptom presentation, as well as treatment response.

THE MUSCULAR IDEAL

As briefly mentioned earlier, the male body ideal typically features a dual focus on a drive for both muscularity and leanness (ie, low body fat).[23] This distinct male ideal offers unique consequences for patterns in ED behaviors and attitudes. For instance, males may be motivated to pursue rigid eating or exercise routines, as well as the use of appearance-enhancing or performance-enhancing drugs (eg, anabolic steroids) to achieve a muscular body idea. Males also endorse a drive for thinness (as females might also report a desire for muscularity) but among males, muscular-oriented disordered eating is considerably more common.[26] A specific pattern of behaviors within muscularity-oriented disordered eating involves what is referred to as "bulking and cutting," and describes an oscillation between pursuit of muscularity and leanness, respectively.[32] During bulking, targeted consumption of protein is typical and often includes somewhat rigid and arbitrary guidelines for the amount, timing, and type of protein consumed.[33,34] Deviation from these rules may cause distress, but it is also during this phase that body image distress related to a desire for leanness may emerge.[26] Henceforth follows the cutting phase, whereby dietary restriction can be extreme, and is typically intended to decrease body fat (ie, improving muscular definition). Cutting may limit muscular development and trigger further body image distress, thereby setting into motion a maladaptive cycle of muscle building and alternating dietary restriction. Although much of the empirical evidence for these practices is nascent, up to 60% of all boys in the United States report purposefully manipulating their diet in striving for greater muscularity,[35] suggesting salient links between muscularity orientation and ED pathology.

Muscle Dysmorphia

Muscle dysmorphia, originally conceptualized as opposite to AN and referred to as "reverse anorexia," was initially identified in a study of male body builders.[36] In a seminal study, some participants displayed similarities to patients with AN, especially related to body image distortion. As would be considered opposite to traditionally internalized body image in AN, core body image distortion in these men manifested as the belief that they were skinny and small, despite being large and muscular. Although preference for a more muscular build may begin at a young age for boys, current average age of onset of muscle dysmorphia occurs in later adolescence.[37] Cognitively, men who experience muscle dysmorphia may have obsessive thoughts about their lack of muscularity, which behaviorally may lead to excessive weight lifting or exercise[23] and rigidity in adhering to a dietary regimen that enhances muscle development.[33,38] Associated with muscle dysmorphia, anabolic steroids are used predominantly by male-identified individuals with muscularity-focused body dissatisfaction,[39] and their use is considerably more common among homosexual male adolescents than those who identify as heterosexual.[40] In DSM-5, muscle dysmorphia is currently classified as a unique body dysmorphic disorder associated with muscularity concerns,[19] although some researchers propose that this pattern of symptoms may more aptly be classified as part of the ED spectrum.[38]

Proposed factors that negatively affect body image among youth and adolescents include media, family, and friends.[41] A recent study of social media use among sexual minority male adults found that higher frequency of use of social media platforms, and particularly those that were body centric in focus (eg, Facebook, Instagram), was associated with greater muscularity-oriented body image concerns and eating pathology.[42] Although this study was conducted among adult participants, its findings are relevant to youth and adolescents who are frequent consumers of social media. Other risks for eating pathology that are evident among sexual minority males are detailed in the next section.

RISK ASSOCIATED WITH SEXUAL ORIENTATION

Over several decades, evidence has accumulated in support of an association between sexual orientation and ED symptoms in adults, particularly in men,[43–47] and in adolescent males.[48–50] In examination of trends over time in eating pathology among adolescent sexual minority subgroups, although notably improved compared with sexual minority females, males continue to report higher prevalence of purging, using diet pills, and fasting to lose weight compared with their heterosexual counterparts.[50] It seems that increased prevalence exists across a variety of ED symptoms; in a recent cohort study in the United Kingdom, at age 14 years, homosexual and bisexual boys reported significantly greater body dissatisfaction than their same-sex heterosexual peers.[49] At this age, sexual minority boys also reported greater dysfunctional eating behaviors compared with their heterosexual peers. At age 16 years, homosexual and bisexual boys had 12.5 times the likelihood of engaging in binge eating as heterosexual boys.[49] In other large community-based studies in the United States, homosexual males[51] and males with same-sex sexual partners[52] reported increased ED symptoms compared with heterosexual males and males with other-sex partners. In a nationally representative cohort of high school students in Norway, male adolescents with same-sex sexual experience were more likely to report bulimic symptoms than those without same-sex sexual experience (estimated 7 times the risk in males with same-sex sexual experience).[53] Taken together, the extant research on models of ED and their intersection with sexual orientation suggest that sexual minority status may be a contributing risk factor for ED among young males.

CLINICAL IMPACT OF A FEMALE-CENTRIC FRAMEWORK OF ASSESSMENT AND TREATMENT

Moving both within and beyond a long history whereby men are consistently marginalized in screening, treatment, and research of EDs, there are several areas that receive the greatest impact from the traditionally held female-centric ED framework. One of these domains is treatment seeking, or what some have referred to as "help seeking."[7] Lack of insight, denial, shame, and secrecy are all factors that have an impact on willingness to seek treatment of EDs across the sexes. However, this influence may be greater among males, given perceived stigma associated with disclosure of mental health issues.[7,54] Further, despite widespread efforts to convey an opposite missive, cultural stereotypes still perpetuate the perception that EDs are typically a female disorder. Stigmatizing beliefs about the presentation of AN among men may contribute to the latency for males to present to treatment. Perhaps as a result of this delay, 50% of male adolescent ED presentations for treatment results in the need for immediate hospitalization.[54] One recent study of adolescent males presenting for treatment found that nearly half had a history of being overweight or obese. Subsequently, the mean percentage of median body mass index in this sample was 88.8%, a value that is in line with other work indicating higher premorbid weights among males compared with females, which likely contributes to a delay in receiving treatment.[55] However, in this study, patients had lost an average of 21.5% of premorbid body weight, consistent with severe malnutrition and presented with significantly dysregulated vital signs.[56] Reducing stigma and improving screening and detection of symptoms consistent with EDs among young males is clearly an important endeavor in future directions of clinician education, particularly within standard pediatric clinical care.

FUTURE DIRECTIONS

Although there is increasing momentum within the field to focus specifically on the screening, assessment, and study of ED presentation among adolescent males, considerable efforts are required to attenuate to the knowledge base within the field, established for EDs among female peers. Toward that end, some specific domains are highlighted whereby targeted research would be optimized. Perhaps the most important of these domains is in the area of improving the tools with which male ED symptom pathology is screened, assessed, and diagnosed. The removal of amenorrhea as a diagnostic criterion for AN within DSM-5 was an important step in improving accuracy in prevalence estimates among boys. However, there is no current diagnostic category that can accommodate inclusion of a muscularity-oriented body image as opposed to a thinness ideal. Given consistent presentation of muscular-oriented body image concerns and related behaviors, this lack of conceptual framework is concerning.[57] Further, evidence suggests that males report less severe overall ED psychopathology compared with females.[17] However, it is likely that much of the gold standard assessments reveal lower scores among boys given a lack of validity and sensitivity within specific items.[15] Given a limited number of studies specific to boys, low sample size in samples of men in mixed-sex trials and assessment methods that retain bias and cull symptoms more specific to females (eg, internalization of a thin ideal),[32,57] developing and testing assessment tools specifically among males is unequivocally essential to future assessment, diagnostic, and treatment endeavors.

Related to current issues with assessment among males is consideration of the age of ED onset among males, because research to date has been conflicting. On the one hand, evaluation of ED symptoms in a large cohort sample suggested that loss of control eating may be nearly twice as common in older boys as in younger boys; concerns about weight and shape also seem to increase substantially from early to late adolescence.[18] However, other work has found that in certain populations, such as sexual minority males, binge eating and purging behaviors were consistently greater than heterosexual peers (aged 12–23 years), across all ages.[58] Early identification of EDs is important across the sexes, but in light of the aforementioned barriers to treatment seeking, earlier efforts to screen and assess boys for ED symptoms should be prioritized. Overall, in most cases, it seems that as male adolescents age, reported cognitive and behavioral ED symptoms seem to worsen, indicating that early intervention is of critical importance.[18]

Most investigations of EDs among adolescent males has been conducted within a western cultural milieu, and overwhelmingly comprised of individuals who identify as white. Thus, future research should include attention to potential differences in risk and ED presentation in males, intersected with cultural and ethnic identification. Some existing literature indicates that non-white boys, and in particular those of Latino and African American identification, demonstrate higher rates of disordered weight control behaviors compared with white or Asian boys.[48,59–61] However, other work found that weight control behavior and concerns were equally or more prevalent among all non-whites, including higher risk among Asian American boys.[58] Overall, there are largely mixed findings in the relationship between ED symptoms and cultural and ethnicity-related factors. Compounding the dearth of methodologically valid assessment tools to index ED symptoms among men, an even greater gap exists surrounding psychometric evaluation of symptoms with cultural sensitivity. Future endeavors should include testing of both existing and to-be-developed indices of ED symptoms across diverse male samples.

Moving beyond screening and assessment efforts, no treatments to date have been tailored to the clinical presentation of boys and tested accordingly. Precision ED treatment of boys should directly address muscularity-oriented body image concerns, potentially minimizing exercise behavior that exacerbates and maintains these symptoms. Further, given the consistent evidence indicating increased risk and severity of ED pathology among sexual minority boys, treatment that specifically addresses a broad spectrum of gender and sexual presentations, including among those who identify as transgender or gender fluid, is necessary. Many current treatment centers with specialty in a higher level of care are unable to admit boys to their service, given logistical issues with housing boys and girls separately, leading to further marginalization and internalized stigma among young men and their families who seek treatment.

SUMMARY

Estimates of prevalence for EDs among youth and adolescent males are likely considerably underestimated. Perpetuation of the perception that EDs are largely a female phenomenon over nearly 5 decades has led to the consistent exclusion of young men from research efforts, and subsequent paucity of understanding and accuracy in classification and assessment. Although increased appreciation of eating and body image concerns among males has been demonstrated, methods of identification, assessment, classification, and treatment specific to male concerns are critically in need of advancement. Particularly as epidemiologic studies indicate that EDs among males are advancing equally or perhaps even more quickly than among females, it is essential that the thinness-oriented body image characteristic of a traditional ED framework be re-evaluated and adjusted. Further, males present with symptoms that are as severe as their female counterparts, indicating that increased awareness and early identification of these disorders among young men is crucial. As screening efforts are honed and stigma is reduced, presentation of males to treatment will also increase. It will be important for clinicians to familiarize themselves with the clinical presentation of EDs among males, as well as to increase education efforts surrounding optimal treatment approaches.

REFERENCES

1. Schaumberg K, Welch E, Breithaupt L, et al. The science behind the academy for eating disorders' nine truths about eating disorders. Eur Eat Disord Rev 2017; 25(6):432–50.
2. Gull W. Anorexia nervosa (apepsia hysterica, anorexia hysterica). Trans Clin Soc London 1874;7:22.
3. Bruch H. Anorexia nervosa in the male. Psychosom Med 1971;33:31–47.
4. Hudson JI, Hiripi E, Pope HG, et al. The prevalence and correlates of eating disorders in the National Comorbidity Survey replication. Biol Psychiatry 2007;61: 349–58.
5. Murray SB, Griffiths S, Mond JM. Evolving eating disorder psycho- pathology: conceptualizing muscularity-oriented disordered eating. Br J Psychiatry 2016; 208:414–5.
6. Mitchison D, Hay P, Slewa-Younan A, et al. The changing demographic profile of eating disorder behaviors in the community. BMC Public Health 2014;14:943.

7. Mitchison D, Mond JM. Epidemiology of eating disorders, eating disordered behaviour, and body image disturbance in males: a narrative review. J Eat Disord 2015;3:20.

8. Woodside DB, Garfinkel PE, Lin E, et al. Comparisons of men with full or partial eating disorders, men without eating disorders, and women with eating disorders in the community. Am J Psychiatry 2001;158(4):570–4.

9. Madden S, Morris A, Zurynski YA, et al. The burden of eating disorders in 5–13-year-old children in Australia. Med J Aust 2009;190:410–4.

10. Nicholls DE, Lynn R, Viner RM. Childhood eating disorders: British national surveillance study. Br J Psychiatry 2011;198:295–301.

11. Eddy KT, Thomas JT, Hastings E, et al. Prevalence of DSM-5 avoidant/restrictive food intake disorder in a pediatric gastroenterology healthcare network. Int J Eat Disord 2014;48:464–70.

12. Field A, Sonneville K, Crosby R, et al. Prospective associations of concerns about physique and the development of obesity, binge drinking, and drug use among adolescent boys and young adult men. JAMA Pediatr 2014;168(1):34–9.

13. Gueguen J, Godart N, Chambry J, et al. Severe anorexia nervosa in men: comparison with severe AN in women and analysis of mortality. Int J Eat Disord 2012;45(4):537–45.

14. Murray SB, Griffiths S, Nagata JM. Community-based eating disorder research in males: a call to action. J Adolesc Health 2018;62(6):649–50.

15. Darcy AM, Doyle AC, Lock J, et al. The eating disorders examination in adolescent males with anorexia nervosa: how does it compare to adolescent females? Int J Eat Disord 2012;45:110–4.

16. Murray SB, Nagata JM, Griffiths S, et al. The enigma of male eating disorders: a critical review and synthesis. Clin Psychol Rev 2017;57:1–11.

17. Smith KE, Mason TB, Murray SB, et al. Clinical norms and sex differences on the Eating Disorder Inventory (EDI) and the Eating Disorder Examination Questionnaire (EDE-Q). Int J Eat Disord 2017;50:769–75.

18. Mond J, Hall A, Bentley C, et al. Eating-disordered behavior in adolescent boys: eating disorder examination questionnaire norms. Int J Eat Disord 2014;47(4):335–41.

19. American Psychiatric Association. Diagnostic and statistical manual of mental disorders. 5th ed. Washington, DC: APA; 2013.

20. Allen KL, Byrne SM, Oddy WH, et al. Early onset binge eating and purging eating disorders: course and outcome in a population-based study of adolescents. J Abnorm Child Psychol 2013;41(7):1083–96.

21. Kjelsås E, Bjørnstrøm C, Götestam KG. Prevalence of eating disorders in female and male adolescents (14–15 years). Eat Behav 2004;5(1):13–25.

22. Smink FR, van Hoeken D, Oldehinkel AJ, et al. Prevalence and severity of DSM-5 eating disorders in a community cohort of adolescents. Int J Eat Disord 2014;47(6):610–9.

23. Pope HG, Phillips KA, Olivardia R. The Adonis complex: the secret crisis of male body obsession. New York: The Free Press; 2000.

24. Goodwin H, Haycraft E, Meyer C. The relationship between compulsive exercise and emotion regulation in adolescents. Br J Health Psychol 2012;17:699–710.

25. Hay P, Girosi F, Mond J. Prevalence and sociodemographic correlates of DSM-5 eating disorders in the Australian population. J Eat Disord 2015;3(1):19.

26. Lavender JM, Brown TA, Murray SB. Men, muscles, and eating disorders: an overview of traditional and muscularity-oriented disordered eating. Cur Psychiatry Rep 2017;19(6):32.

27. Pila E, Mond JM, Griffiths S, et al. A thematic content analysis of #cheatmeal images on social media: characterizing an emerging trend. Int J Eat Disord 2017; 50(6):698–706.
28. Cooney M, Lieberman M, Guimond T, et al. Clinical and psychological features of children and adolescents diagnosed with avoidant/restrictive food intake disorder in a tertiary care eating disorder program. J Adolesc Health 2017;60(2):S46.
29. Fishe MM, Rosen DS, Ornstein RM, et al. Characteristics of avoidant/restrictive food intake disorder in children and adolescents: a "new disorder" in DSM-5. J Adolesc Health 2014;55(1):49–52.
30. Nicely TA, Lane-Loney S, Masciulli E, et al. Prevalence and characteristics of avoidant/restrictive food intake disorder in a cohort of young patients in day treatment for eating disorders. J Eat Disord 2014;2:21.
31. Norris M, Norris L, Katzman DK. Change is never easy, but is it possible: reflections on avoidant/restrictive food intake disorder two years after its introduction in the DSM-5. J Adolesc Health 2015;57:8–9.
32. Griffiths S, Murray SB, Touyz SW. Disordered eating and the muscular ideal. J Eat Disord 2013;1:15.
33. Mosley PE. Bigorexia: bodybuilding and muscle dysmorphia. Eur Eat Disord Rev 2009;17(3):191–8.
34. Murray SB, Rieger E, Touyz SW. Muscle dysmorphia symptomatology during a period of religious fasting: a case report. Eur Eat Disord Rev 2011;19:162–8.
35. Eisenberg MA, Wall M, Nuemark-Sztainer D. Muscle-enhancing behaviors among adolescent girls and boys. Pediatrics 2012;130:1019–26.
36. Pope HG Jr, Katz DL, Hudson JI. Anorexia nervosa and "reverse anorexia" among 108 male bodybuilders. Compr Psychiatry 1993;34(6):406–9.
37. Olivardia R. Mirror, mirror on the wall, who's the largest of them all? The features and phenomenology of muscle dysmorphia. Harv Rev Psychiatry 2001;9:245–59.
38. Murray SB, Rieger E, Touyz SW, et al. Muscle dysmorphia and the DSM-V conundrum: where does it belong? A review paper. Int J Eat Disord 2010;43:483–91.
39. Pope HG, Kanayama G, Hudson JI. Risk factors for illicit anabolic-androgenic steroid use in male weightlifters: a cross-sectional cohort study. Biol Psychiatry 2012;71:254–61.
40. Blashill AJ, Calzo JP, Griffiths S, et al. Anabolic steroid misuse among US adolescent boys: disparities by sexual orientation and race/ethnicity. Am J Public Health 2017;107:319–21.
41. Ricciardelli LA, McCabe MP, Banfield S. Body image and body change methods in adolescent boys: role of parents, friends, and the media. J Psychosom Res 2000;49:189–97.
42. Griffiths S, Murray SB, Krug I, et al. The contribution of social media to body dissatisfaction, eating disorder symptoms, and anabolic steroid use among sexual minority men. Cyberpsychol Behav Soc Netw 2018;21(3):149–56.
43. Beren SE, Hayden HA, Wilfley DE, et al. The influence of sexual orientation on body dissatisfaction in adult men and women. Int J Eat Disord 1996;20(2): 135–41.
44. Carlat DJ, Camargo CA Jr. Review of bulimia nervosa in males. Am J Psychiatry 1991;148(7):831–43.
45. Feldman MB, Meyer IH. Eating disorders in diverse lesbian, gay, and bisexual populations. Int J Eat Disord 2007;40(3):218–26.
46. Frederick DA, Essayli JH. Male body image: the roles of sexual orientation and body mass index across five national US Studies. Psychol Men Masc 2016; 17(4):336.

47. Russell CJ, Keel PK. Homosexuality as a specific risk factor for eating disorders in men. Int J Eat Disord 2002;31:300–6.
48. Austin SB, Nelson LA, Birkett MA, et al. Eating disorder symptoms and obesity at the intersections of gender, ethnicity, and sexual orientation in US high school students. Am J Public Health 2013;103(2):e16–22.
49. Calzo JP, Austin SB, Micali N. Sexual orientation disparities in eating disorder symptoms among adolescent boys and girls in the UK. Eur Child Adolesc Psychiatry 2018;27(11):1483–90.
50. Watson RJ, Adjei J, Saewyc E, et al. Trends and disparities in disordered eating among heterosexual and sexual minority adolescents. Int J Eat Disord 2017; 50(1):22–31.
51. French SA, Story M, Remafedi G, et al. Sexual orientation and prevalence of body dissatisfaction and eating disordered behaviors: A. Int J Eat Disord 1996;19(2): 119–26.
52. Ackard DM, Fedio G, Neumark-Sztainer D, et al. Factors associated with disordered eating among sexually active adolescent males: gender and number of sexual partners. Psychosom Med 2008;70:232–8.
53. Wichstrøm L. Sexual orientation as a risk factor for bulimic symptoms. Int J Eat Disord 2006;39(6):448–53.
54. Griffiths S, Mond JM, Murray SB, et al. Young peoples' stigmatizing attitudes and beliefs about anorexia nervosa and muscle dysmorphia. Int J Eat Disord 2014; 47(2):189–95.
55. Raevuori A, Keski-Rahkonen A, Hoek H. A review of eating disorders in males. Curr Opin Psychiatry 2014;27:426e30.
56. Vo M, Lau J, Rubinstein M. Eating disorders in adolescent and young adult males: presenting characteristics. J Adolesc Health 2016;59:397–400.
57. Murray SB, Griffiths S, Hazery L, et al. Go big or go home: a thematic content analysis of pro-muscularity websites. Body Image 2016;16:17–20.
58. Neumark-Sztainer D, Croll J, Story M, et al. Ethnic/racial differences in weight-related concerns and behaviors among adolescent girls and boys: findings from Project EAT. J Psychosom Res 2002;53(5):963–74.
59. Field AE, Colditz GA, Peterson KE. Racial/ethnic and gender differences in concern with weight and in bulimic behaviors among adolescents. Obes Res 1997;5(5):447–54.
60. Johnson WG, Rohan KJ, Kirk AA. Prevalence and correlates of binge eating in white and African American adolescents. Eat Behav 2002;3(2):179–89.
61. Nicdao EG, Hong S, Takeuchi DT. Prevalence and correlates of eating disorders among Asian Americans: results from the National Latino and Asian American Study. Int J Eat Disord 2007;40(suppl):S22–6.

Use of Technology in the Assessment and Treatment of Eating Disorders in Youth

Shiri Sadeh-Sharvit, PhD[a,b],*

KEYWORDS

- Blended therapy • Eating disorders • Mobile health • Online treatment • Self-help
- Smartphone applications • Youth

KEY POINTS

- Digital technologies complement existing methods of treatment delivery as they facilitate and augment established best practices.
- Technology could help overcome common barriers in eating disorder treatment, including cost, access, stigma, the paucity of professionals trained in empirically supported interventions, and the limited appeal of such treatment.
- Online programs and smartphone apps allow sharing of real-time monitoring of symptoms with the treating clinicians, making the intervention more focused and accurate.
- Telemedicine and telepsychology are integrated into existing services for eating disorders and increase the relevancy and immediacy of treatment.
- Digital self-help programs have been found to be effective and accepted by clients with eating disorders and/or their families.

INTRODUCTION

Smartphone applications (apps), Internet programs, wearable devices, and related technologies have dramatically changed the way people perceive and learn about the world and about themselves, interact with each other, and make changes in their daily lives. Digital and ubiquitous technologies can facilitate and augment many aspects of clinical practice and are especially poised to attract youth experiencing mental health difficulties.[1] One group of illnesses often beginning during childhood and early adolescence is eating disorders, which are highly debilitating and life-threatening, with a potentially chronic course. Eating disorders impede functions

Conflict of Interest: The author reports no conflicts of interest.
[a] Baruch Ivcher School of Psychology, Interdisciplinary Center, Kanfei Nesharim 1, Herzliya 4610101, Israel; [b] Center for m²Health, Palo Alto University, Palo Alto, CA, USA
* Baruch Ivcher School of Psychology, Interdisciplinary Center, Kanfei Nesharim 1, Herzliya 4610101, Israel.
E-mail address: sshiri@idc.ac.il

that are keys to childhood and adolescent health, namely physical growth, social interactions, and academic performance. However, because eating disorders are also highly stigmatized, and affordable and accessible treatment by providers trained in empirically supported methods is scarce, many individuals do not receive the treatment they need. Technological tools are especially poised to appear attractive to youth with eating disorders: young people are considered early adopters of new technologies, and they report a preference for communicating via text messaging rather than phone calls, are more inclined to use apps and record their data online, and have increased media literacy.[2,3] Furthermore, technologies that connect the provider and the client could diminish the imbalance of power that is often inherent to the treatment relationship, particularly in treatment of eating disorders in children and adolescents.

The promising benefits of digital tools for youth with eating disorders and their capabilities could be demonstrated using a model for integrating technology into clinical practice (**Fig. 1**). This model illuminates how incorporating digital services in all steps of mental health care assessment and delivery has the potential to facilitate clinical insights, augment treatment effects, provide useful resources to supplement learning new skills, and understand risk and maintenance factors associated with target symptoms.

A MODEL FOR INTEGRATING TECHNOLOGY IN CLINICAL PRACTICE

To understand how technology aids and expands the diagnosis and treatment of eating disorders, permit a walk through the common tasks providers endeavor to complete when working with a client reporting eating disorder symptoms. Online screening for self-assessment could benefit thousands of individuals who are unsure whether their symptoms merit an intervention. Some digital tools are also available for clinicians assessing symptoms of treatment-seeking individuals. Furthermore, online programs and smartphone apps are particularly important because they can provide real-time monitoring and assessment. They can also inform the provider whether the intervention is effective in reducing target symptoms. Digital tools are often used in teletherapy, that is, providing mental health services remotely, via text messaging (during or following treatment) or using a Web-conferencing platform to deliver treatment rather than via a face-to-face meeting. Technology can be leveraged to provide psychoeducation and help the clients practice skills, as part of the current intervention or

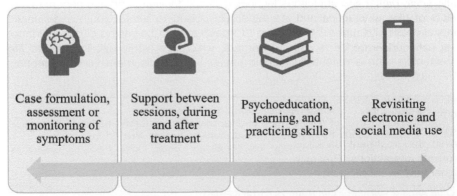

Fig. 1. Integrating technology into the assessment and treatment of eating disorders in youth.

separately. Finally, inquiry into patients' use and consumption of electronic and social media, online video games, and video streaming services is a key to identifying and targeting behaviors that could impede the patients' use of the intervention.

DIGITAL TOOLS FOR ASSESSING AND MONITORING EATING DISORDER SYMPTOMS

Online screening tools that are data driven can help individuals assess their current symptoms by providing personalized feedback and triage to appropriate resources, as needed. Online screening is likely the first step in identifying possible cases in the community and reducing the burden of eating disorders.[4] However, screens that detect cases are not also suitable to identify at-risk behaviors.[5] For instance, the Stanford–Washington University Eating Disorder Screen screening tool assigns respondents into *no-risk*, *low-risk*, *high-risk*, and *present eating disorder* categories and provides tailored feedback.[6,7] This tool is suitable to respondents 13 years of age and older and is presently available via the National Eating Disorder Association Web site, at www.nationaleatingdisorders.org/screening-tool. When clients arrive for the initial evaluation, a digital version of a *Diagnostic and Statistical Manual of Mental Disorders* (5th ed; *DSM-5*)[8] interview can assist the interviewer in reaching the most suitable diagnosis. The Eating Disorder Assessment for *DSM-5* (EDA-5) is a semistructured interview that aims to help clinicians in assessing whether the client meets criteria for a DSM-5 eating disorder.[9] The EDA-5 is freely available at https://eda5.org.

Once a diagnosis is reached, the client and the therapist both depend on an understanding of symptom severity, contexts for problematic cognitions, and emotions and behaviors that trigger and maintain the eating disorder. Smartphone apps are superior to the old pen-and-paper food logs because they allow greater real-time, private monitoring. Some apps, such as Recovery Record, have features providing cell phone notifications, graphs of target behaviors over a distinct duration of time (ie, the past month or week), and sharing of data with the clinician, should the user choose to do this.[10] Digital technologies seem to attract a sizable group of users who do not present to face-to-face treatment. A recent study on Recovery Record users found that despite having eating disorder symptoms for more than 9 years, on average, about half of these users reported never having received specialized treatment of those symptoms.[11] Hence, specialized apps may be the only platform some people would use, particularly if they believe other forms of treatment are currently unavailable for them. Of note, wearable devices and smartphone apps that provide passive or active self-monitoring could be misused by individuals with eating disorders. For instance, the lion's share of users of wearable fitness trackers and apps that serve as calorie counters experienced more disordered eating and dietary restraint and perceived them as detrimental to their well-being and reinforcing their eating disorder.[12,13]

SUPPORT BETWEEN SESSIONS

Interventions featuring the delivery of psychological and medical services using telecommunication technologies for clients with eating disorders are mushrooming.[14,15] Telepsychology services can be either synchronous or asynchronous, intertwined within the treatment package, or represent more spontaneous forms of client-provider interactions. Presently, expectations for health providers' availability are higher than ever before.[16]

Text and e-mail messaging with clients has become more mainstream within medical services, even in more traditional approaches to psychotherapy.[17] The more medical problems the individual experiences, the more they are likely to send and receive messages from their physician, nurse, or health promotion organization.[18] Cognitive-behavioral and dialectical-behavioral treatments may include routine e-mail coaching as part of the intervention; however, in general, no clear guidelines have been proposed.[19] A text-based maintenance intervention for individuals with bulimia nervosa (BN) and bulimic symptoms demonstrated higher remission rates. In this model, participants sent text updates on their condition to their therapist for 16 weeks following their discharge from inpatient treatment and received tailored feedback.[20]

Clinicians who have been trained in empirically supported approaches are scarce. Commute time to treatment, affordability, and waitlists in certain clinics often hinder many potential consumers from meeting a therapist face to face. Evidence indicates that the treatment can be delivered remotely, using Web-conferencing services, with few changes to the intervention and with adequate efficacy.[21] Furthermore, technology allows for more convenient scheduling of sessions, with little travel time, and flexibility in scheduling sessions. A pilot study testing family-based treatment of anorexia nervosa (AN) delivered via Web-conferencing yielded significant weight restoration and a decrease in cognitions associated with eating and comorbid psychopathologies.[22] Another study, a randomized controlled trial (RCT) of group cognitive-behavioral therapy for BN, delivered either face to face or via chat, found that the former version produced quicker improvement in target symptoms (ie, abstinence from binge-eating and purging); however, by the 12-month follow-up, both methods of delivery were equally effective.[23]

One caveat to using these services is that they need to be encrypted (or compliant with the Health Insurance Portability and Accountability Act, or HIPPA, in the United States), using digital platforms that require paid subscription from private users. In addition, therapists are permitted to practice where they are licensed, and all parties to the Web conversation likely need access to high-speed Internet or mobile data coverage as well as privacy while communicating remotely. Nevertheless, safety, privacy, and confidentiality considerations all must be addressed before the first teletherapy session.[24]

TECHNOLOGY TO PROVIDE TREATMENT COMPONENTS OR SUBSTITUTES

Use of technology can be especially useful in delivering components of an intervention or substituting it altogether. For instance, the therapist can refer families to viewing psychoeducational material on YouTube or specialized Web sites for individuals with eating disorders that offer information that is sound, evidence supported, and reliable, such as that of Maudsley Parents (www.maudsleyparents.org) or Project HEAL (www.theprojectheal.org). Furthermore, recent implementations of virtual reality tools in treatment were found to augment the intervention's effect on reducing body image dissatisfaction.[25]

Because of barriers such as stigma, access, cost, and lack of trained practitioners, most individuals with eating disorders worldwide are unable to present to treatment. Therefore, digital self-help bridges this gap between need and available programs. These self-help programs typically consist of segments accessed via the Internet or an app (called "sessions") that translate previously book-based self-help materials into video and audio files as well as practice exercises. The self-help can be either "pure," that is, the individual is expected to independently work through materials, or "guided," supplemented with the option to communicate with a facilitator who provides online coaching and personalizes the program to the individual user.[26] In general, online programs for individuals with eating disorders have been proven effective in decreasing risk factors for eating disorders and symptoms, including reducing body dissatisfaction, thin-ideal internalization, weight and shape concerns, caloric restriction, binge-eating, and purging.[27]

Of these digitally delivered models, it appears that guided self-help for the treatment of eating disorders has done the most to capitalize on the benefits of technology in designing interventions that are feasible, acceptable to mental health consumers, and associated with improved outcomes. For instance, a guided self-help program for adolescents with AN applied the principles of family-based treatment.[28] Over the course of 12 weeks, parents were granted access to videos, reading materials, and a parent discussion forum. Parents were also asked to self-monitor the strategies they viewed as effective in their renourishment efforts. In addition, the parents received short weekly consultations with an experienced clinician via a Web-conferencing platform or the telephone. Findings indicated that this self-help program facilitated weight restoration and reduced eating and cooccurring psychopathology, and that its effects were sustainable over time.[28] Other online guided self-help programs specifically designed for individuals with clinical or subthreshold eating disorders have reduced shape and weight concerns, eating disorders symptoms for participants whose symptoms were initially greater elevated.[29,30] These interventions also incorporate the support of facilitators who personalized the program for individual users, to make it more relevant to the user's difficulties and dilemmas when applying the intervention to their lives.[31] However, most guided programs have not yet made the necessary adaptations for minors with eating disorders, such as attaining parental consent and exploring collaborations with family members and educators.

REVIEWING THE CLIENT'S USE OF ELECTRONIC AND SOCIAL MEDIA

Youth Internet habits worry parents, pediatricians, clinicians, educators, and other stakeholders. Although the American Academy of Pediatrics recommends parents set clear limits to screen time and social media use,[32] most children and adolescents accept the ideas of constant online interconnection, social media presence, and screen time as given; however, the long-term impacts on their brains and mental health are still undetermined.[33] Web sites promoting harmful and misleading ideas, such as proanorexia and probulimia sites and those using hashtags, such as *#fitspration*, often operate with the facade of prohealth and supportive resources, reinforce symptom continuance, and hinder help-seeking behaviors and recovery, which makes them confusing and possibly dangerous to young people.[34] It appears that the internalization of the thin ideal increases young women's vulnerability to feeling more negative about their bodies, following media exposure.[35] However, although communicating with clients about their electronic and social media use patterns appears likely to be beneficial, studies indicate most clinicians fail to include these topics in their routine assessment and treatment. For instance, individuals who received treatment of their eating disorders in a group setting reported interacting on social media with treatment peers and/or organizations related to eating disorders. Those who reported greater social comparisons to their social media friends also reported greater eating disorder psychopathology. However, only a fifth of participants in this study have ever been asked by a therapist about their social media use patterns.[36]

In contrast to the troubling data on how electronic and social media fuel eating disorders, promising evidence indicates that teaching adolescent girls to consume media critically is likely to reduce disordered eating and negative body image.[35] Social and electronic media literacy interventions train participants in appraising media content through identifying and challenging harmful messages appearing in these outlets.[37] Therefore, these interventions may provide teens with context and skills that potentially inoculate them for harmful impacts of such media. Social media can also serve as a vehicle for empowerment, information, healthful advice, and support and operate in concert with young people's preferred means of mental health self-help and support.[38]

CHALLENGES IN USING TECHNOLOGY WITH YOUTH AFFECTED WITH EATING DISORDERS

The many benefits technology provides for assessing and treating children and adolescents with eating disorders are not without shortcomings. Although parents (or other guardians, as appropriate) are legally responsible for monitoring their children's access and use of Internet assessments, smartphone apps, and online social networks, a clinician choosing to incorporate technology into their practice must obtain parental consent in addition to the young individual's assent.[39] Therapists delivering treatment remotely should treat collaboration and routine check-ins with parents, as well as parental counseling sessions, as an imminent part of the intervention, similarly to what they would do in a face-to-face delivery. Likewise, collaborating with physicians, dietitians, teachers, coaches, and other significant individuals in the young person's life remains an essential part of treatment, even when it is delivered remotely.[40]

Another important prerequisite to practicing with digital tools is educating the client about confidentiality and privacy and their limitations. Text and e-mail messages might be intercepted by others who were not intended to read the correspondence. Practitioners should make sure that the tools they use are not only encrypted (for instance, Web sites whose address begins with "https:") but also compliant with the HIPPA and other federal and state laws. Furthermore, integrating technology into existing services inevitably requires more therapist time and possibly paid subscription to these services and therefore may result in increased fees, particularly for services that are yet to be reimbursed by insurance companies. Greater time expenditure may result in "workplace telepressure," a phenomenon associated with greater psychological detachment, higher levels of burnout, and poorer sleep quality.[41]

One may argue that current treatment should focus on deterring youth from online communication and prevent additional use of electronic and social media; inviting children and adolescents to include technology in their treatment has the potential to reinforce fewer face-to-face interactions and increase youth's vulnerability to harmful online content. However, data from RCTs testing the integration of digital resources into health care delivery have been positive and promising in terms of long-term adaptation, maintenance of recovery, and greater media literacy.[27,42,43] Another caveat to developing additional self-help resources is that insurance companies might recommend them to clients because they are low cost and reduce or eliminate face-to-face treatments, whose effectiveness is superior to that of self-help programs. Similarly, apps and self-help programs might hinder the user from seeking higher levels of care, when appropriate. Furthermore, there is a significant research-to-practice gap in the study of technologies to aid clients with additional feeding and eating disorders, such as avoidant/restrictive food intake disorder or pica, who could benefit from such services.

SUMMARY

Consumer demand for digitally enabled clinical services is growing faster than the professional response.[44] Although some of the tools described in this article are relatively new and innovative, these fresh methods complement and extend clinicians' already-established best practices of mental health care and service delivery. The digital tools available in the eating disorders field capitalize on empirically supported models, namely, cognitive-behavioral and family-based therapies. In addition, most aforementioned technologies have proven feasible, acceptable, and effective when implemented with individuals with eating disorders. Nevertheless, ethical and professional guidelines have yet to be established, and many clinicians think they need help in becoming more competent in technology use and blended therapy models. Because eating disorders are serious and sometimes life-threatening disorders that usually onset during childhood and adolescence,[8] using technology, which appears to have a positive impact on treatment efficacy, symptom reduction, and better adaptation, could help us provide better services to our clients in the journey to help them live healthier, more rewarding lives.

REFERENCES

1. Mohr DC, Riper H, Schueller SM. A solution-focused research approach to achieve an implementable revolution in digital mental health. JAMA Psychiatry 2018;75(2):113–4.
2. Schickedanz A, Huang D, Lopez A, et al. Access, interest, and attitudes toward electronic communication for health care among patients in the medical safety net. J Gen Intern Med 2013;28(7):914–20.
3. Anderson M. Technology device ownership: 2015. Washington, DC: Pew Research Center; 2015.
4. Carlson LE, Waller A, Groff SL, et al. Online screening for distress, the 6th vital sign, in newly diagnosed oncology outpatients: randomised controlled trial of computerised vs personalised triage. Br J Cancer 2012;107(4):617–25.
5. Jacobi C, Abascal L, Taylor CB. Screening for eating disorders and high-risk behavior: caution. Int J Eat Disord 2004;36(3):280–95.
6. Graham AK, Trockel M, Weisman H, et al. A screening tool for detecting eating disorder risk and diagnostic symptoms among college-age women. J Am Coll Health 2019;67(4):357–66.
7. Fitzsimmons-Craft EE, Balantekin KN, Graham AK, et al. Results of disseminating an online screen for eating disorders across the US: reach, respondent characteristics, and unmet treatment need. Int J Eat Disord 2019;52(6):721–9.
8. American Psychiatric Association. Diagnostic and statistical manual of mental disorders. DSM-5. Washington, DC: APA Press; 2013.
9. Sysko R, Glasofer DR, Hildebrandt T, et al. The eating disorder assessment for DSM-5 (EDA-5): development and validation of a structured interview for feeding and eating disorders. Int J Eat Disord 2015;48(5):452–63.
10. Tregarthen JP, Lock J, Darcy AM. Development of a smartphone application for eating disorder self-monitoring. Int J Eat Disord 2015;48(7):972–82.
11. Sadeh-Sharvit S, Kim JP, Darcy AM, et al. Subgrouping the users of a specialized app for eating disorders. Eat Disord 2018;26(4):361–72.
12. Levinson CA, Fewell L, Brosof LC. My Fitness Pal calorie tracker usage in the eating disorders. Eat Behav 2017;27:14–6.
13. Simpson CC, Mazzeo SE. Calorie counting and fitness tracking technology: associations with eating disorder symptomatology. Eat Behav 2017;26:89–92.
14. American Psychological Association. Guidelines for the practice of telepsychology 2013. Available at: https://www.apa.org/practice/guidelines/telepsychology.aspx.

15. Shingleton RM, Richards LK, Thompson-Brenner H. Using technology within the treatment of eating disorders: a clinical practice review. Psychotherapy 2013; 50(4):576–82.
16. Topol E. The patient will see you now: the future of medicine is in your hands. New York, NY: Basic Books; 2015.
17. Sucala M, Schnur JB, Brackman EH, et al. Clinicians' attitudes toward therapeutic alliance in E-therapy. J Gen Psychol 2013;140(4):282–93.
18. Newhouse N, Lupiáñez-Villanueva F, Codagnone C, et al. Patient use of email for health care communication purposes across 14 European countries: an analysis of users according to demographic and health-related factors. J Med Internet Res 2015;17(3):e58.
19. Morin J-FG, Harris M, Conrod PJ. A review of CBT treatments for substance use disorders. New York: Oxford Handbooks; 2017.
20. Bauer S, Okon E, Meermann R, et al. Technology-enhanced maintenance of treatment gains in eating disorders: efficacy of an intervention delivered via text messaging. J Consult Clin Psychol 2012;80(4):700–6.
21. Morland LA, Greene CJ, Rosen CS, et al. Telehealth and eHealth interventions for posttraumatic stress disorder. Curr Opin Psychol 2017;14:102–8.
22. Anderson KE, Byrne CE, Crosby RD, et al. Utilizing Telehealth to deliver family-based treatment for adolescent anorexia nervosa. Int J Eat Disord 2017;50(10): 1235–8.
23. Zerwas SC, Watson HJ, Hofmeier SM, et al. CBT4BN: a randomized controlled trial of online chat and face-to-face group therapy for bulimia nervosa. Psychother Psychosom 2017;86(1):47–53.
24. Drum KB, Littleton HL. Therapeutic boundaries in telepsychology: unique issues and best practice recommendations. Prof Psychol Res Pr 2014;45(5):309.
25. Marco JH, Perpiñá C, Botella C. Effectiveness of cognitive behavioral therapy supported by virtual reality in the treatment of body image in eating disorders: one year follow-up. Psychiatry Res 2013;209(3):619–25.
26. National Collaborating Centre for Mental Health. Common mental health disorders: identification and pathways to care. Chesham, UK: RCPsych Publications; 2011.
27. Melioli T, Bauer S, Franko DL, et al. Reducing eating disorder symptoms and risk factors using the internet: a meta-analytic review. Int J Eat Disord 2016;49(1): 19–31.
28. Lock J, Darcy A, Fitzpatrick KK, et al. Parental guided self-help family based treatment for adolescents with anorexia nervosa: a feasibility study. Int J Eat Disord 2017;50(9):1104–8.
29. Kass AE, Trockel M, Safer DL, et al. Internet-based preventive intervention for reducing eating disorder risk: a randomized controlled trial comparing guided with unguided self-help. Behav Res Ther 2014;63:90–8.
30. Taylor CB, Kass AE, Trockel M, et al. Reducing eating disorder onset in a very high risk sample with significant comorbid depression: a randomized controlled trial. J Consult Clin Psychol 2016;84(5):402.
31. Carrard I, Fernandez-Aranda F, Lam T, et al. Evaluation of a guided internet self-treatment programme for bulimia nervosa in several European countries. Eur Eat Disord Rev 2011;19(2):138–49.
32. Council on Communications and Media. Media use in school-aged children and adolescents. Pediatrics 2016;138(5):e20162592.
33. Kaliebe K, Weigle P. Child psychiatry in the age of the internet. Child Adolesc Psychiatr Clin N Am 2018;27(2):xiii–xv.

34. Rouleau CR, von Ranson KM. Potential risks of pro-eating disorder websites. Clin Psychol Rev 2011;31(4):525–31.
35. Bair CE, Kelly NR, Serdar KL, et al. Does the Internet function like magazines? An exploration of image-focused media, eating pathology, and body dissatisfaction. Eat Behav 2012;13(4):398–401.
36. Saffran K, Fitzsimmons-Craft EE, Kass AE, et al. Facebook usage among those who have received treatment for an eating disorder in a group setting. Int J Eat Disord 2016;49(8):764–77.
37. Wade TD, Wilksch SM, Paxton SJ, et al. Do universal media literacy programs have an effect on weight and shape concern by influencing media internalization? Int J Eat Disord 2017;50(7):731–8.
38. Kendal S, Kirk S, Elvey R, et al. How a moderated online discussion forum facilitates support for young people with eating disorders. Health Expect 2017;20(1):98–111.
39. Harris J, Porcellato L. Opt-out parental consent in online surveys: ethical considerations. J Empir Res Hum Res Ethics 2018;13(3):223–9.
40. Ackard DM, Neumark-Sztainer D. Health care information sources for adolescents: age and gender differences on use, concerns, and needs. J Adolesc Health 2001;29(3):170–6.
41. Barber LK, Santuzzi AM. Please respond ASAP: workplace telepressure and employee recovery. J Occup Health Psychol 2015;20(2):172–89.
42. Halliwell E, Easun A, Harcourt D. Body dissatisfaction: can a short media literacy message reduce negative media exposure effects amongst adolescent girls? Br J Health Psychol 2011;16(2):396–403.
43. Slone NC, Reese RJ, McClellan MJ. Telepsychology outcome research with children and adolescents: a review of the literature. Psychol Serv 2012;9(3):272.
44. Mattison M. Social work practice in the digital age: therapeutic e-mail as a direct practice methodology. Soc Work 2012;57(3):249–58.

UNITED STATES POSTAL SERVICE ® Statement of Ownership, Management, and Circulation (All Periodicals Publications Except Requester Publications)

1. Publication Title	2. Publication Number	3. Filing Date
CHILD AND ADOLESCENT PSYCHIATRIC CLINICS OF NORTH AMERICA	011 – 368	9/18/2019

4. Issue Frequency	5. Number of Issues Published Annually	6. Annual Subscription Price
JAN, APR, JUL, OCT	4	$335.00

7. Complete Mailing Address of Known Office of Publication (Not printer) (Street, city, county, state, and ZIP+4®)

ELSEVIER INC.
230 Park Avenue, Suite 800
New York, NY 10169

Contact Person
STEPHEN R. BUSHING
Telephone (include area code)
215-239-3688

8. Complete Mailing Address of Headquarters or General Business Office of Publisher (Not printer)

ELSEVIER INC.
230 Park Avenue, Suite 800
New York, NY 10169

9. Full Names and Complete Mailing Addresses of Publisher, Editor, and Managing Editor (Do not leave blank)

Publisher (Name and complete mailing address)

TAYLOR BALL, ELSEVIER INC.
1600 JOHN F KENNEDY BLVD. SUITE 1800
PHILADELPHIA, PA 19103-2899

Editor (Name and complete mailing address)

LAUREN BOYLE, ELSEVIER INC.
1600 JOHN F KENNEDY BLVD. SUITE 1800
PHILADELPHIA, PA 19103-2899

Managing Editor (Name and complete mailing address)

PATRICK MANLEY, ELSEVIER INC.
1600 JOHN F KENNEDY BLVD. SUITE 1800
PHILADELPHIA, PA 19103-2899

10. Owner (Do not leave blank. If the publication is owned by a corporation, give the name and address of the corporation immediately followed by the names and addresses of all stockholders owning or holding 1 percent or more of the total amount of stock. If not owned by a corporation, give the names and addresses of the individual owners. If owned by a partnership or other unincorporated firm, give its name and address as well as those of each individual owner. If the publication is published by a nonprofit organization, give its name and address.)

Full Name	Complete Mailing Address
WHOLLY OWNED SUBSIDIARY OF REED/ELSEVIER, US HOLDINGS	1600 JOHN F KENNEDY BLVD. SUITE 1800 PHILADELPHIA, PA 19103-2899

11. Known Bondholders, Mortgagees, and Other Security Holders Owning or Holding 1 Percent or More of Total Amount of Bonds, Mortgages, or Other Securities. If none, check box. → ☐ None

Full Name	Complete Mailing Address
N/A	

12. Tax Status (For completion by nonprofit organizations authorized to mail at nonprofit rates) (Check one)
The purpose, function, and nonprofit status of this organization and the exempt status for federal income tax purposes:
☒ Has Not Changed During Preceding 12 Months
☐ Has Changed During Preceding 12 Months (Publisher must submit explanation of change with this statement)

PS Form 3526, July 2014 (Page 1 of 4 (see instructions page 4)) PSN 7530-01-000-9931 PRIVACY NOTICE: See our privacy policy on www.usps.com

---

13. Publication Title	14. Issue Date for Circulation Data Below
CHILD AND ADOLESCENT PSYCHIATRIC CLINICS OF NORTH AMERICA	JULY 2019

15. Extent and Nature of Circulation			Average No. Copies Each Issue During Preceding 12 Months	No. Copies of Single Issue Published Nearest to Filing Date
a. Total Number of Copies (Net press run)			154	155
b. Paid Circulation (By Mail and Outside the Mail)	(1)	Mailed Outside-County Paid Subscriptions Stated on PS Form 3541 (Include paid distribution above nominal rate, advertiser's proof copies, and exchange copies)	80	90
	(2)	Mailed In-County Paid Subscriptions Stated on PS Form 3541 (Include paid distribution above nominal rate, advertiser's proof copies, and exchange copies)	0	0
	(3)	Paid Distribution Outside the Mails Including Sales Through Dealers and Carriers, Street Vendors, Counter Sales, and Other Paid Distribution Outside USPS®	22	30
	(4)	Paid Distribution by Other Classes of Mail Through the USPS (e.g., First-Class Mail®)	0	0
c. Total Paid Distribution (Sum of 15b (1), (2), (3), and (4))			102	120
d. Free or Nominal Rate Distribution (By Mail and Outside the Mail)	(1)	Free or Nominal Rate Outside-County Copies Included on PS Form 3541	40	22
	(2)	Free or Nominal Rate In-County Copies Included on PS Form 3541	0	0
	(3)	Free or Nominal Rate Copies Mailed at Other Classes Through the USPS (e.g., First-Class Mail)	0	0
	(4)	Free or Nominal Rate Distribution Outside the Mail (Carriers or other means)	0	0
e. Total Free or Nominal Rate Distribution (Sum of 15d (1), (2), (3) and (4))			40	22
f. Total Distribution (Sum of 15c and 15e)			142	142
g. Copies not Distributed (See Instructions to Publishers #4 (page #3))			12	13
h. Total (Sum of 15f and g)			154	155
i. Percent Paid (15c divided by 15f times 100)			71.83%	84.51%

* If you are claiming electronic copies, go to line 16 on page 3. If you are not claiming electronic copies, skip to line 17 on page 3.

PS Form 3526, July 2014 (Page 2 of 4)

16. Electronic Copy Circulation	Average No. Copies Each Issue During Preceding 12 Months	No. Copies of Single Issue Published Nearest to Filing Date
a. Paid Electronic Copies	▲	
b. Total Paid Print Copies (Line 15c) + Paid Electronic Copies (Line 16a)	▲	
c. Total Print Distribution (Line 15f) + Paid Electronic Copies (Line 16a)	▲	
d. Percent Paid (Both Print & Electronic Copies) (16b divided by 16c × 100)	▲	

☒ I certify that 50% of all my distributed copies (electronic and print) are paid above a nominal price.

17. Publication of Statement of Ownership

☒ If the publication is a general publication, publication of this statement is required. Will be printed ☐ Publication not required.
in the OCTOBER 2019 issue of this publication.

18. Signature and Title of Editor, Publisher, Business Manager or Owner		Date
STEPHEN R. BUSHING – INVENTORY DISTRIBUTION CONTROL MANAGER	*Stephen R. Bushing*	9/18/2019

I certify that all information furnished on this form is true and complete. I understand that anyone who furnishes false or misleading information on this form or who omits material or information requested on the form may be subject to criminal sanctions (including fines and imprisonment) and/or civil sanctions (including civil penalties).

PS Form 3526, July 2014 (Page 3 of 4) PRIVACY NOTICE: See our privacy policy on www.usps.com

Moving?

Make sure your subscription moves with you!

To notify us of your new address, find your **Clinics Account Number** (located on your mailing label above your name), and contact customer service at:

Email: journalscustomerservice-usa@elsevier.com

800-654-2452 (subscribers in the U.S. & Canada)
314-447-8871 (subscribers outside of the U.S. & Canada)

Fax number: 314-447-8029

Elsevier Health Sciences Division
Subscription Customer Service
3251 Riverport Lane
Maryland Heights, MO 63043

*To ensure uninterrupted delivery of your subscription, please notify us at least 4 weeks in advance of move.

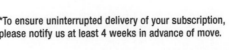
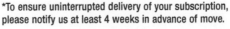

Printed and bound by CPI Group (UK) Ltd, Croydon, CR0 4YY

03/10/2024

01040480-0014